Sphere Fields, Qi Gong and AIDS

MINGGUO CHO

ISBN-10: 1523719435
ISBN-13: 978-1523719433

DEDICATION

This book is dedicated to AIDS patients and their doctors; homosexuals and their relatives; religious people and atheists; legislators, lawyers, and judges; pharmaceutical companies; and insurance companies.

CONTENTS

Acknowledgments   i

Preface   1

Foreword   6

1   Background   Cell Magnetic Fields: A Healing System   9

2   Structure of the Human Body   15

3   What is AIDS?   29

4   Definition of Homosexuality   31

5   Etiology and Contagion of AIDS   39

6   How to Prevent AIDS Contagion   46

7   How to Cure (Heal) AIDS   49

8   Advice for Homosexual and AIDS Patients   66

9   Key Points in the Practice of Qi Gong   69

10   Conclusion   75

11   A Few Cases of Non-medical Healing Under the
Guidance of the Author (1988)   81

12   A Few Cases of Medical Healing Under the
Treatment by the Author (includes AIDS patient,
LUPUS patient up to 2013)   93

13   Functions and Utilization of Qi Gong   113

14   Questions and Answers Readers May Have   122

Appendix A   AIDS Update News   176

Appendix B   Falun Gong Brochure   177

About the Author

ACKNOWLEDGMENTS

A special thanks to those teachers who had taught me Qi Gong: Dr. Wen-You Hshieh (Tai-Chi Chuan); Mr. Timothy Hsieh (WuSan Chu Ni-Chong Qi Gong); Dr. Ching-Tse Lee (Zhen Man Ching Nine-Turn Qi Gong); Master Hong-ShenSen (Tai-Chi Five Elements Gong); Mr. Fong Liang (Inner Power One Finger Zen); and Master Hong-Chi Lee (Fa Lun Da Fa). Also, I have to give special thanks to my uncle—Mr. Binsen Lin, who gave me a gift—a Chinese medical textbook (*Yi Chong Gyn Ghien*). With this book, I solved the whole picture of herbal treatments. I extend a great thanks to my relatives who helped me in the past thirty years with this research and book.

PREFACE

During the writing of this book, the author experienced a great deal of apprehension. The ideas in this book have been on his mind for about six years (1982-1988), but the writing process has been slow because of having to work to support himself and his family.

The basic ideas are simple, yet they include almost everything. In fact, they can explain phenomena which were thought to be miracles or scientific mysteries. The grasp of the theory is so awesome as to be frightening, so the author has challenged himself about it again and again, wishing it was wrong. But, as more and more information came out, his convictions became stronger. The incredible has become reasonable and there are fewer actual miracles.

Continually it came to his mind; he became obsessed with these ideas. They intruded upon his consciousness very often while working or reading, and pushed him to write them down as soon as possible.

Also, a good friend died of cancer, and there have been a number of famous people who died of A.I.D.S. All these have made him feel guilty that he didn't tell the world about his idea and that those who died couldn't be cured, especially when his American friend died of kidney cancer. In the beginning, when the author heard his friend was sick, he already had envisioned that it was cancer. The author said to his friend's wife Judy, "If it is cancer, don't allow him to have surgery, maybe we can find some other way to heal it." Yet, maybe because the author is not a known authority, his warning was not heeded. His friend had surgery and died within three months. Chinese doctors say that, when people get cancer, the earlier the surgery the earlier the death. That was true before 1988. This case and cases of so many other people have made the author very sad because they didn't have this medical concept that the author presents in this book. It should be a generally popular concept and it should help people get the right treatment in order to recover from illness. The author wants to publish this book to help people as soon as possible, in the hope that it can bring the proper medical concept to the public. Furthermore, the book seeks to solve our many medical problems by gathering the efforts of different specialists.

After you read this book, you will find that there are many small things mentioned which are worth years of study. Time is running out for many patients who are very ill. The author is willing to discuss with any patient their illness and recommend types of treatment.

The author expresses a sincere thanks to the following people: Dr. Ching-Tse Lee and Mr. Timothy Hsieh who taught him Qi Gong. Without them, he would not have his ideas about Qi. Mrs. Helen Marmor, NBC's former executive producer, helped to edit his original manuscript. Mrs. Mary Ann Carroll helped him to translate the manuscript from Chinese to English and typed it from the rough draft. Also, the author has to thank Donald MacLaren for his help editing and preparing the book.

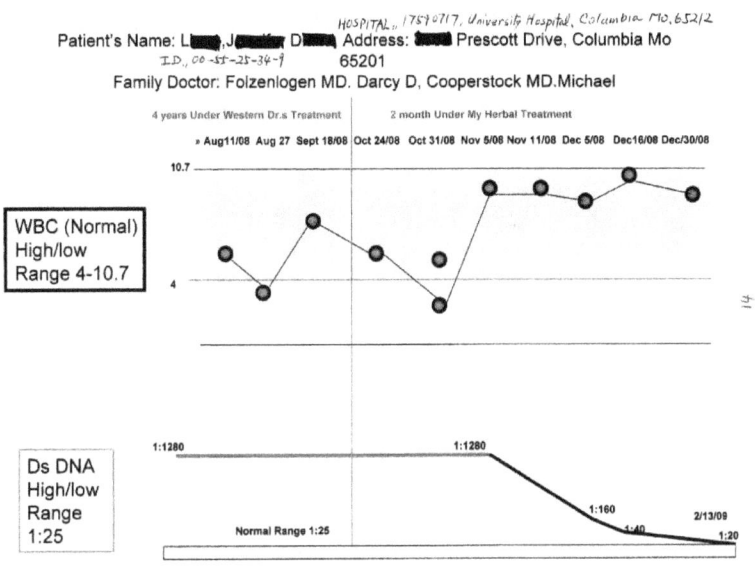

Patient's Name: L___, J___ D___ Address: ___ Prescott Drive, Columbia Mo
HOSPITAL// 1757 0717, University Hospital, Columbia MO, 65212
I.D., 00 -55 -25 -34 -9   65201
Family Doctor: Folzenlogen MD. Darcy D, Cooperstock MD.Michael

4 years Under Western Dr.s Treatment | 2 month Under My Herbal Treatment

» Aug11/08 Aug 27 Sept 18/08 | Oct 24/08 Oct 31/08 Nov 5/08 Nov 11/08 Dec 5/08 Dec16/08 Dec/30/08

WBC (Normal) High/low Range 4-10.7

10.7
4

Ds DNA High/low Range 1:25

1:1280   1:1280
Normal Range 1:25   1:160   2/13/09
1:40   1:20

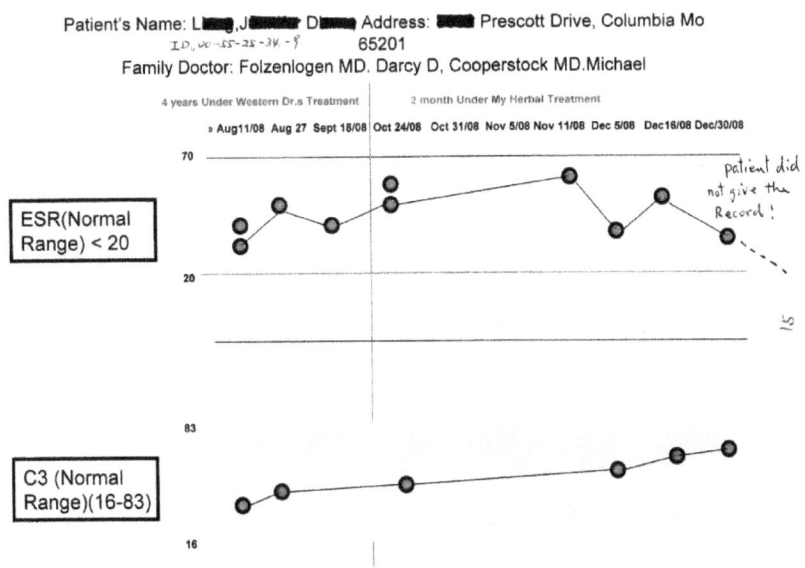

Patient's Name: L___, J___ D___ Address: ___ Prescott Drive, Columbia Mo
I.D., 00 -55 -25 -34 -9   65201
Family Doctor: Folzenlogen MD. Darcy D, Cooperstock MD.Michael

4 years Under Western Dr.s Treatment | 2 month Under My Herbal Treatment

» Aug11/08 Aug 27 Sept 18/08 | Oct 24/08 Oct 31/08 Nov 5/08 Nov 11/08 Dec 5/08 Dec16/08 Dec/30/08

ESR(Normal Range) < 20

70
20

patient did
not give the
Record !

C3 (Normal Range)(16-83)

83
16

3

Patient's Name: L███,J███ D███, Address: ███ Prescott Drive, Columbia Mo
ID: 00-55-25-34-9   65201
Family Doctor: Folzenlogen MD. Darcy D, Cooperstock MD.Michael

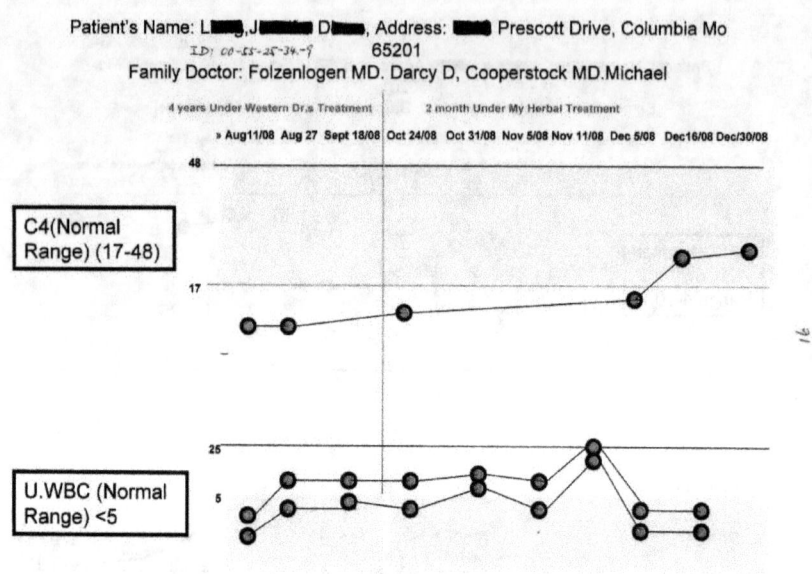

Patient's Name: L███,J███ D███, Address: ███ Prescott Drive, Columbia Mo
ID, 00-55-25-34-9   65201
Family Doctor: Folzenlogen MD. Darcy D, Cooperstock MD.Michael

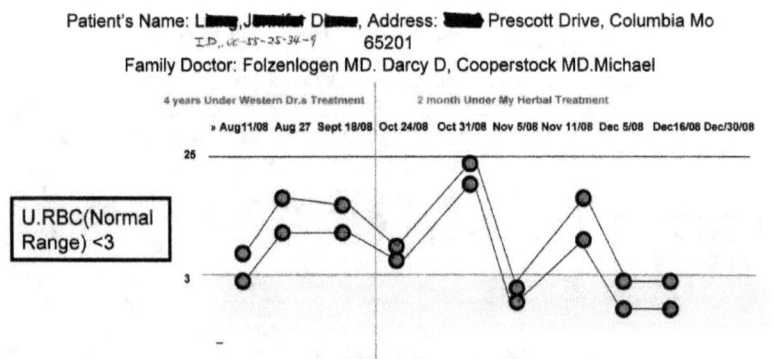

4

This to prove that even the Nephritis is not problem for the Author.

Patient's Name:Chiang,▮▮▮▮..Hospital: Mount Sinai Hospital , one Gustane Ley

ID, 2828981   Place ,N.Y.N.Y.10029

Diagnosis : Grade IV LUPUS , NEPHRITIS - S(4) , Post Bronchoscopy , Post Pericardio Centesis

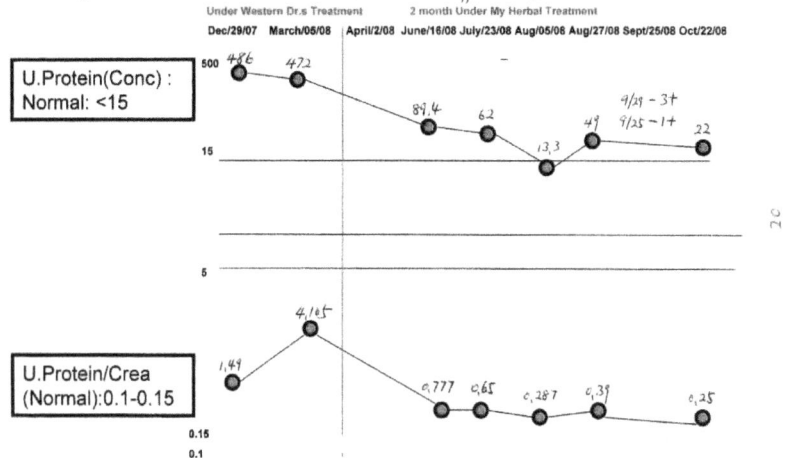

Patient's Name:Chiang,▮▮▮..Hospital: Mount Sinai Hospital , one Gustane Ley

I.D. 2828981   Place ,N.Y.N.Y.10029

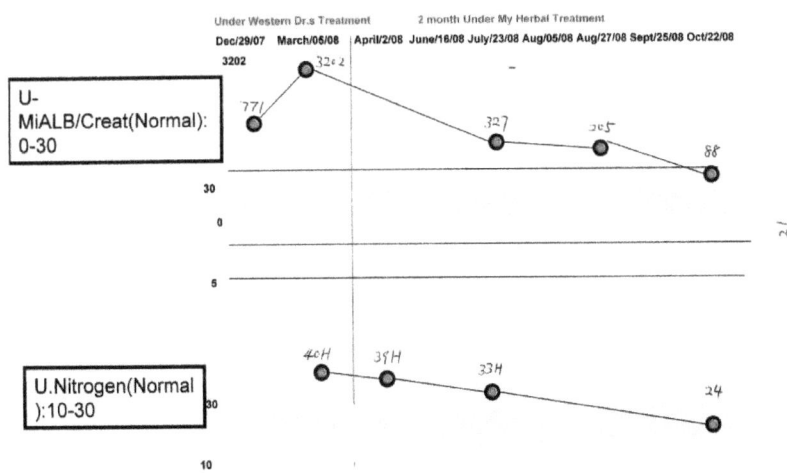

5

FOREWORD

This book draft was finished twenty-five years ago. However, after the author showed it to ten of his Ph.D. friends, they all said that without experimental evidence or case studies, any theory means nothing in the medical world. Also, there was a problem since the author had no medical background. (But, today the author has been proved with medical evidence that he is superior to medical specialists.)

So this draft has been sitting in the file since they made their comments.

Now in 2014, it has been twenty-five years since the author has solved the most mysterious disease—LUPUS (This will be developed in another book later). If the reader would like to check, the reader can check the following court case: (only the court case can show that the author did not lie.)

Attorney General of Missouri, Jefferson City 65102

Attorney General: CHRIS KOSTER: (573)-751-3321

Complaint No. CF-2009-05653   Date: July, 2009

The LUPUS Patient: Ms. L.J.D.   ID: 00-55-25-34-9

Hospital: 17590717, University Hospital. Columbia, Missouri 65212

Sick since February, 2004   Diagnosis as LUPUS, nephritis

The patient was given up by the hospital on the middle of October, 2008 after four and a half years of treatment.

The author took over and cured her LUPUS, but the cure did not include Nephritis (the damaged organ) within three months with herbal medicine.

WBC 4.9 → 8.3, ESR 61 → 28, C3 46 → 62, C4 10 → 24

U.WBC 5 ~ 8 → 0 ~ 3, URBC 20 ~ 25 → 0 ~ 3, ds DNA 1:1280 → 1:20 (90 days) and after that, within month became normal without herbal medicine.

And the author was in New York City and never saw the patient before and after. Then, the author is not a day dreamer. The witness Dr. Cooper Stock is Dean of the Hospital. Telephone: 573-882-4141/Fax: 573-884-4277.

Besides this example, the author predicted that there would be different types of viruses to appear, like the flu virus. This is proved today. Unfortunately, "AIDS patients should be divided into four classes to study" has not been aware by doctors so far. That is why the real cause could not be found. These four types are: (1) One with AIDS symptoms, but no virus; (2) one with symptoms also with virus. These are still two kinds of patients who should be divided: (2.a) he is a gay man receiver or (2.b) not and (4) one with virus, but no symptoms that lead to different results, even with the same new medicine treatment: some patients seem under control and improving, but some are totally out of control. Doctors could not understand because they did not divide the patients into the four groups as the author said. And the major reason is the patients' sexual histories were confidential. So, no doctors could do this kind of study and research.

Today, to legalize homosexual marriages is almost done (personally, the author is for the legalization because that makes the medical study more clear and easy. However, the sexual ID is yet not cleared: male, who like the female only, male sees male as female, male sees male as female sees male, female sees female as male sees female.). But the religious people are upset about having no scientific reasons to support the Bible's saying to be against homosexual marriages. So does the parent. And the most horrible fact is that the homosexual couples (gay men) who claim to love each other, but they did not know during lovemaking one is killing the other.

The author is an architectural engineer (art and engineer

training). That is why he is curious and interested in different sexual activity, but because he is cautious he also did study. That makes this book complete. And after twenty-five years, the author from semi-pro became superior to the ordinary medical professional, so he thinks it is time to publish this book.

CHAPTER 1

BACKGROUND
CELL MAGNETIC FIELDS: A HEALING SYSTEM

One dreaded shadow hanging over humanity is that of AIDS. No one knows how or where the disease began. There are theories and speculation as to its origins, including other continents and other animals. Nor has anyone developed methods of treatment for this twentieth-century scourge. Medication is still only in the research and testing phase.

So far, our limited knowledge includes the following facts:

- Children can inherit AIDS in utero by direct infection from the mother's blood supply.
- The virus can be transmitted by transfusion.
- The virus can be transmitted by certain kinds of sexual contact through body fluids.

The fact that the incidence of AIDS is widespread and still growing is undeniable. It is also undeniable that all the efforts of science so far to deal with a cure have been futile. It is for this reason that we must re-examine our approach and methods.

This book is not designed to be a textbook when it was written, but today should be the most important guide for everyone, including the medical community. The author was not a medical pro (before 1989), but rather an engineer with a lifelong interest in the study of Eastern and Western philosophies and science. He has come upon a system of integrating various phenomena already known in large part, but never heretofore connected.

Note: Now the author is proved superior to the medical specialist in many diseases (2014) for such diseases as lupus and mesothelioma. Those not proved include Alzheimer's, MS (multiple sclerosis), and cancers.

Conventional science begins with presumptions and proceeds to develop proof or a theory to support these preconceptions. The system is:

Assumption – Model – Proof – Theory

For example, Avogadro's Hypothesis, a theory in physics, was postulated in 1811, but it was not until 1858 when an Italian chemist, Stanislao Cannizzaro, built a chemical logic model upon this law and then the law was accepted.

Thus, we are not able to overcome the problems of dealing with the newly developed disease such as AIDS because we are still trying to use our previously held, primarily Western-developed concepts. Scientists are constrained by the narrow range of chemical and medical knowledge which is familiar to them.

New understanding would become apparent if the medical specialists were to look toward neglected historical sources—the knowledge contained in ancient wisdom that is usually rejected by modern scientists because these scientists cannot explain such phenomena. We are talking about truths known for thousands of years and hinted at in writings that have lasted for all these centuries. They can be found in the Bible, Buddhism, Zen, the study of herbal medicine in China, Egypt, or India and in the principles of acupuncture, now becoming a "legitimate" science.

Rather than ignoring, dismissing or disparaging the insights of the scientists, we should actively seek them out and include them in our range of study. If they can achieve the necessary open-mindedness, the scientists can find themselves able to treat or heal a variety of difficult diseases, such as cancer and AIDS. The author has already proved that within twenty-five years effort he really could cure many incurable diseases easily, based on those books that were published thousands of years ago.

Because this new approach is so broadly-based, touching upon a wide range of disciplines, and because the author lacks credentials in the medical field, he offers this book in the hope that the public, patients, and medical specialists will explore the ideas outlined herein. By so doing, the new theory, employing the ancient principles of Qi Gong, will be proved to be correct, enabling society to solve a number of medical and scientific problems.

Today, all the scientists studying AIDS take tissue samples from the patient's body for testing. Even so, how and where the first AIDS case started they cannot offer an answer.

It's like putting out fires without identifying their original causes or at least changing a faulty wiring system that could lead to a fire.

Here are a few conclusions which will be explained in later chapters.

1...The AIDS virus develops (originally) in rectal fissures resulting from anal intercourse. This practice, primarily in male homosexual relationships, damages the human **magnetic field**, causing the human body cells to change their characteristic composition, similar to the cellular process in which magnetic iron changes to steel. In the human body, the virus thus produced damages all the cells' magnetic fields. (See questions and answers in the last chapter: Question 1.)

2...The condom may protect a person from contagion from another person's body fluid, but it cannot avoid or prevent damage to a human body's magnetic field from anal intercourse of two male homosexuals. The virus can be produced as a result of the damaged magnetic field even when a condom is used. (See questions and answers in the last chapter: Question 2.)

3...The invasion of the AIDS virus into the blood stream and thence into the cellular structure destroys the magnetic field throughout the body. In other words, life power is diminished and then destroyed. (See questions and answers in the last chapter: Question 1.)

4...AIDS beginning and contagion:
  (a) The virus develops because the homosexuals' anal intercourse makes only the receiver's body cells change their material and become or produce the virus. However, what frequency and/or duration of anal intercourse will cause or produce the virus the author cannot answer, as this cannot be tested, for obvious reasons.
  (b) Because the body cells which lost the magnetic field already are damaged or destroyed, they transfer the virus through kissing, injection, or by prenatal infection. However, how much of these it takes to do serious damage or make the virus grow and spread also needs to be studied. The author believes that all kinds of body fluids influences will be different, depending on the amount of infectious material and the circumstances or conditions at the time of contact.

5...AIDS should be curable as follows.

   (a) By stopping anal intercourse, people can avoid damaging the human body's magnetic field directly. (See questions and answers in the last chapter: Question 2.)

   (b) Take herbs or foods that can help refuel the Qi or life power. Herbs such as ginseng are very powerful.

   (c) Learn and practice Qi Gong, which has to do with inner power. (Describe Qi Gong Why is it special to someone's health? Yoga also helps to reduce stress, but no mention is made of yoga. (–Explained later in this book: last chapter, Question 7.)

   (d) Develop and use new health technology. Perhaps the modern medical industry will develop a new machine that can strengthen the human body's magnetic field, doing what Qi Gong does for the human body. This machine would need to be more efficient than Qi Gong, especially for those who cannot practice Qi Gong by themselves. (See questions and answers in the last chapter - Question #8.)

6...Definition of death. (Is the definition of death needed? Question 10: It is known that good nutrition, exercise, and reducing stress may reduce the chances of an early death (Question 11).

   (a) Death occurs when life power in a human body is used up and cannot be refueled.

   (b) Death occurs when the head has been separated from the body or one of the six major organs (brain, heart, liver, lung, kidney, and pancreas) can no longer use the life power and ceases to function. When the life power's regeneration system is short in one part, the result is physical death.

The lack of scientific, medical or Chinese literature supporting these ideas is completely lacking. (See questions and answers in the last chapters.) (Question 12)

Chapter (end): Questions and Answers (See Chapter 14)

#1 AIDS is known to be caused by a virus. It has been photographed and identified. Magnetic fields may not explain a virus-caused disease.

#2 Anal intercourse has been only one source of AIDS transmission. AIDS can also be transmitted between heterosexual couples, one of whom has the AIDS virus.

#3 Vaginal intercourse or oral sex has nothing to do with magnetic fields?

#4 Condoms cannot protect the magnetic field? There is no scientific evidence about magnetic fields. The body has electrical fields as evidenced by the use of electrodes in medical tests.

#5 There is too much emphasis on the unproven magnetic fields. If they are proven, list the scientific research that proves the importance of the magnetic fields.

#6 Stopping anal intercourse alone cannot stop the spread of AIDS.

#7 There needs to be scientific evidence that Qi Gong helps to heal. Why is it special to someone's health? **Yoga** also helps to reduce stress, but no mention is made of yoga.

#8 Can a machine be developed to be the cells' magnetic fields?

#9 It has already been suggested that people can wear small magnets to help their health. What about this type of preventative therapy?

#10 Is the definition of death needed?

#11 It is already known that good nutrition, exercise, and reducing stress may reduce the chances of an early death.

#12 The lack of scientific, medical or Chinese literature supporting these ideas is completely lacking.

CHAPTER 2

STRUCTURE OF THE HUMAN BODY

Before we can discuss all the ideas mentioned in the previous chapter, it would be helpful to review the human body structure. However, when we talk about body structure, it's also necessary to know Qi Gong. No matter what background you come from, if you don't know Qi Gong, it will be very difficult to understand what is being proposed here.

It is fortunate that the study of Qi Gong is not that difficult to learn, especially if you study with a Qi Gong master for three months or use a videotape from the Qi Gong study center (check the online Yellow Pages or Google search) and practice every day by yourself for three months. It is not recommended to practice without a teacher because you may make a mistake in practicing resulting in damage to your body. The damage may be difficult to heal since this kind of injury is totally different from the healing theory of Western doctors.

For example, prostate disease or cancer is caused mostly by a clot of "Qi" and blood mixed in the prostate. The readers need to learn how to lead Qi out of the prostate. Then, most of the time the prostate's problems should be gone. This experience the author tried and it resulted in his healing. The method is easy: just stand with legs open, shoulders wide, a little kneel down, and relax the muscles. Then switch the weight from left to right and turn the body right to the end. Then, let the body turn back naturally and switch the weight from right to left, and turn to the left as far as possible. By the sequence of breathing, continue for about 30 minutes (at least) at a time. Do this technique two times a day. Continue for about four weeks. The prostate problems will be gone and healed. (Note: the author was born in 1948 and is still healthy.)

Pretty soon, you will learn the first level of Qi Gong. From that level, you will know where the many acupuncture points are located and how acupuncture techniques were developed.

Moreover, you will find out what is Qi or life power, and that Qi should be in the most position in our body's anatomy. Unfortunately, it has been totally ignores and disparaged by the modern Western doctors. Nevertheless, in ancient China, it was an aphorism that a doctor who does not know Qi is unqualified to be a doctor, but can only be a nurse.

That means, if a doctor does not know what Qi is and its importance and functions in our body, then the doctor is totally unqualified to talk about curing or healing. Even today, the Chinese still think the same way. That is why it is necessary to call this to the attention of all Western doctors.

Also, Western scientists should spend at least three months practicing Qi Gong one to two hours a day to understand what Qi is and the function of Qi. Then, anatomy can be perfectly understood.

Now, assuming that you have already learned Qi Gong and practiced three months, you will most likely be able to sense a Qi moving in your body. More specifically, this Qi is moving along a definite path. The Qi's moving path and direction are the same in everyone's body and go only in one direction along the highway nets (meridians and vessels). (Only one direction may not make sense. Explained better in the last chapter.) The Qi starts from a sphere field, a point about 2~3" below the navel and about 2~3" deep, circulates through the whole body, and returns to the sphere field again.

Sphere Fields. Some translate this to hypogastrium. But that is not meaningful, although pointing to the location is 2-3 inches below the belly button and 2-3 inches deep. That is the place Qi (life energy) enters and leaves. After practicing for a long time, the Qi gathers here and will grow and become more solid like a pearl. The people called this Dan. I translate this as sphere. The location was called Dan Tien. I call it Sphere Field, which means this location is where a pearl can be raised just like plants are raised on a farm.

However, according to *Medical Textbook Golden Rules* page 842, Sphere Field (Dan Tien) in women is uterus and in man it is seminal vesicle: The reason is while in practicing, after three months, usually he will feel the pulse pumping in the area 2 to 3 inches below the belly button and 1 to 2 inches deep, so we called it the "Dan Tien," but actually that is the feeling only, the same as the acupuncture points whose each points connect to the different organs or parts of the body.

What is Qi and what is its function?

First of all, let's compare an automobile, which is made by man, and an animal (man, bird, fish, or horse), which is in nature. Let us study the differences between them.

Our breathing system can be compared to the automobile's carburetor. When the air and the fuel intake screw is too loose or two tight, it will influence the engine's pumping faster or slower. When you try to run faster or slower, you need to adjust your breathing to match your speed and then you can run longer.

Furthermore, if you turn the screw totally tight or totally loose, the engine will stop. That does not mean the engine is now junk. In the same way, a person who is temporarily drowned or suffocated does not mean the person is dead. Theoretically, this kind of "death" could be cured within a short period of time, such as 24 hours. (24 hours seems too long to be resuscitated?—Explained later in this book – Question #38.)

The author has found in a Chinese medical book how to cure this kind of apparent death. As long as the "dead body" still keeps at least a little life energy in the body, that apparent death should be curable.

A human heart is like a car's motor; the skin, kidney and lung are all kinds of filters; the skin also has another function like a radiator; the digestive system is like a small fuel factory like Mobil or Exxon in our body so we can change oil into gasoline to be used.

Anyway, for all kinds of automobile parts, in our body you may find a similarly functioning organ system. There is one important organ system that has not been mentioned in our human anatomy. People seldom think about the anatomy. That constitutes our human body's battery—and where it hides in our anatomy. Is it our brain? No. Our brain is only a complete auto-control computer, but through our nervous system, without a doubt, is a perfect electrical system. There must be a battery existing somewhere in our body. That is also in animal bodies which is why animals also can be treated by acupuncture.

The flow of Qi starts from the sphere field, goes down through the genitals, through the rectum, then up through the spine to the top of the head, then through the center of the forehead, between the eyes, center of the nose, mouth, throat, chest, navel, and back to the sphere field, in a circular path.

This major loop the Chinese call the small universal loop.

It's the major magnetic line, like going from the automobile battery's positive terminal, through the starter and ignition coil, then distributor, then ignition, then grounding, then back to the battery's negative terminal—the motor's electrical cycle.

Of course, besides this major flow, there are many more in the Qi's flow system.

SEE ILLUSTRATIONS THAT FOLLOW

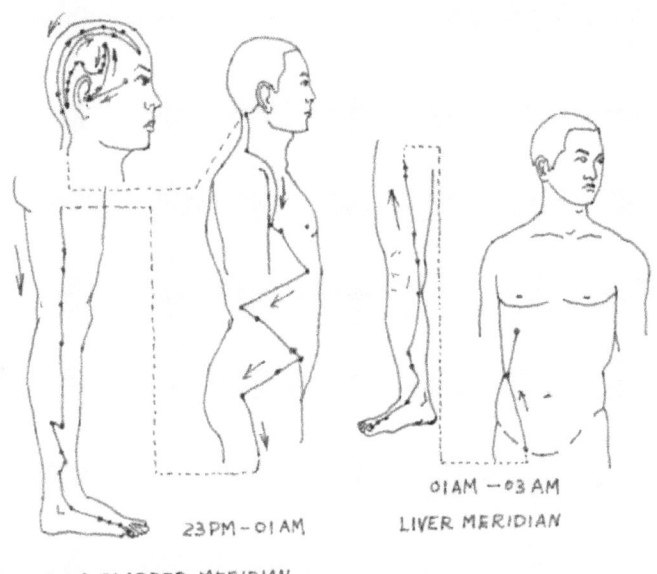

01AM — 03 AM
LIVER MERIDIAN

23PM — 01AM

GALL BLADDER MERIDIAN

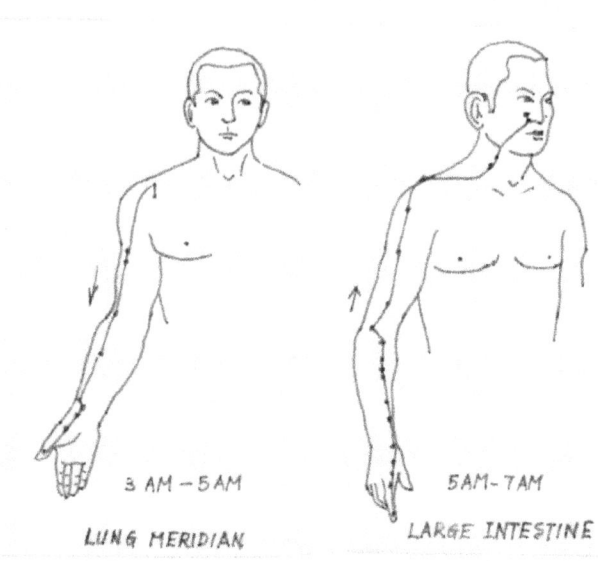

3 AM — 5AM

LUNG MERIDIAN

5AM — 7AM

LARGE INTESTINE

Figure 1A

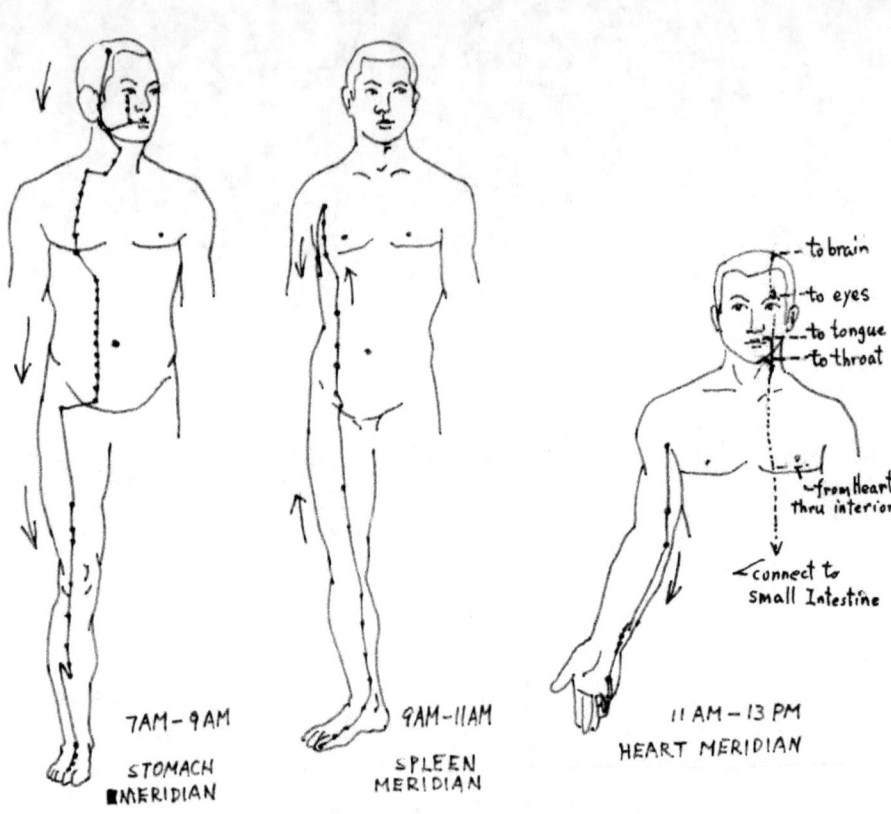

Figure 2B

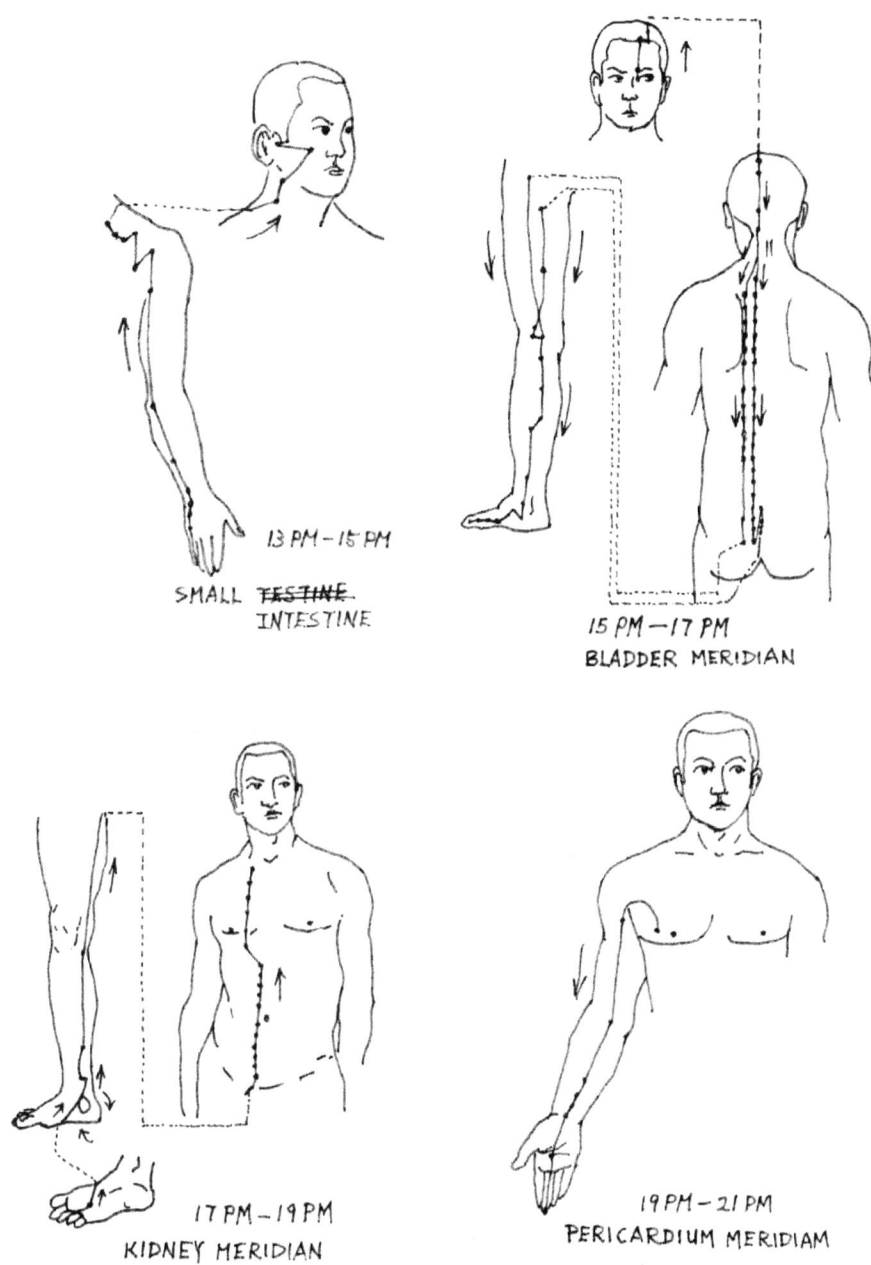

13 PM – 15 PM
SMALL ~~TESTINE~~ INTESTINE

15 PM – 17 PM
BLADDER MERIDIAN

17 PM – 19 PM
KIDNEY MERIDIAN

19 PM – 21 PM
PERICARDIUM MERIDIAM

Figure 3C

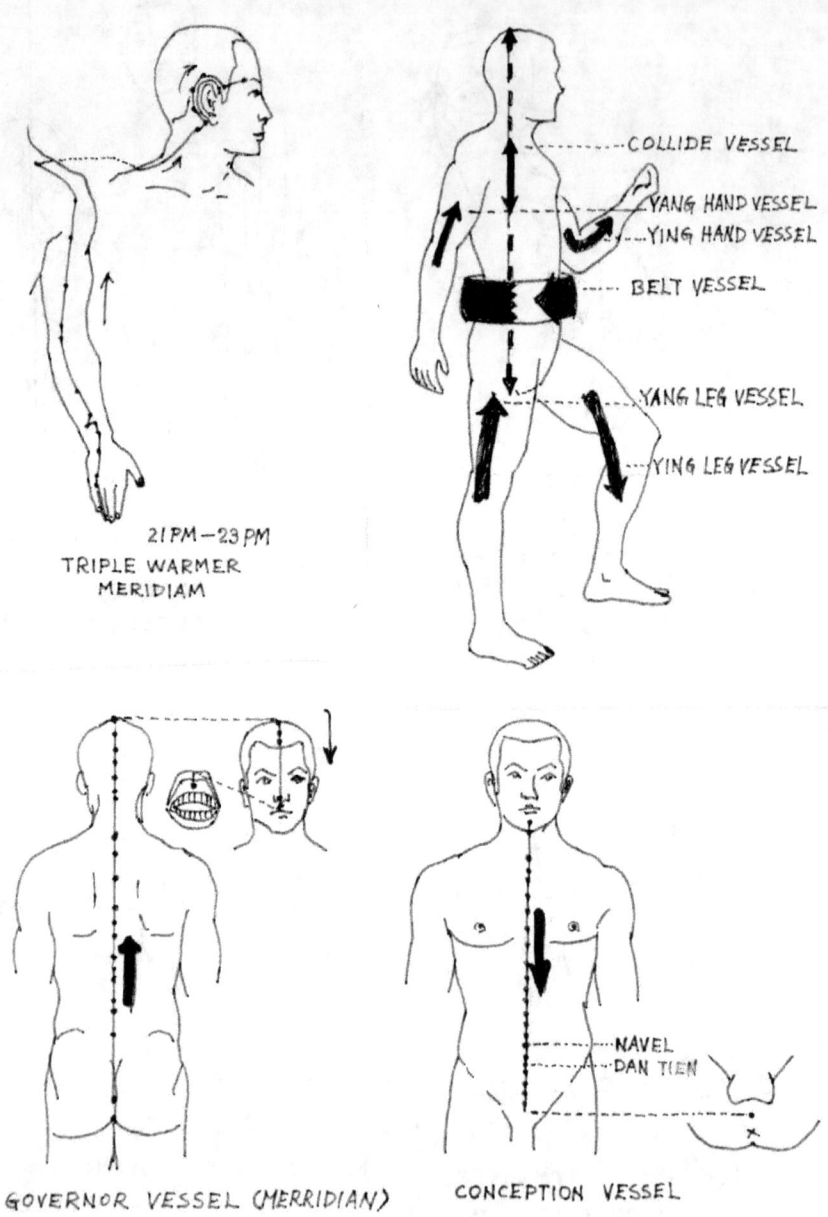

21PM – 23PM
TRIPLE WARMER
MERIDIAM

COLLIDE VESSEL
YANG HAND VESSEL
YING HAND VESSEL
BELT VESSEL
YANG LEG VESSEL
YING LEG VESSEL

NAVEL
DAN TIEN

GOVERNOR VESSEL (MERRIDIAN)   CONCEPTION VESSEL

Figure 4D

When we discuss this, it is apparent that many people cannot wait to criticize the concept.

Typical comments include:

"The electrical system is not the loop system but the nerve system." (Blood has a loop system, but nerves in the body do not loop.) If this idea is correct, then what could the Qi's loop system be? (Can it be proven there is a Qi or that the Qi is a loop? – Question #13)

Note: the nerves do loop.

Why, if for thousands of years the Chinese medical system and Qi Gong already built up a perfect theory, couldn't it be accepted by Western medical specialists? (Qi sounds more like a philosophy rather than a science – Question #14.)

Note: from practice "Yin Diau Gong" Qi really can be measured.

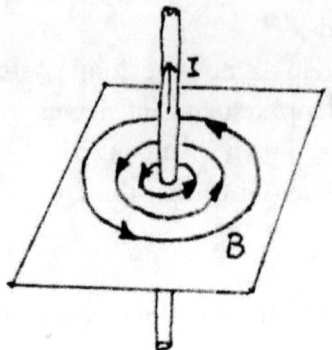

Perspective View

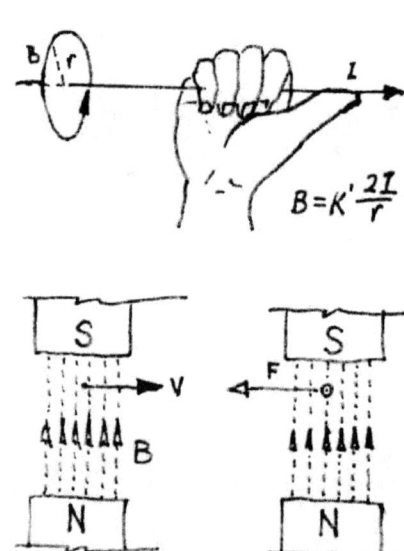

$$B = K' \frac{2I}{r}$$

Figure 5 Author's Notes: Magnetic Fields

Faraday's Right Hand Rule

Top illustration:
Magnetic field surrounding a long straight wire.

Middle illustration: The fingers of the right hand represent the direction of the field, if the thumb is pointed in the direction of the conventional (positive) current.

Right-hand rule for field surrounding long straight wire.
  a...Conductor moving to the right, cutting across a magnetic field.
  b...Lenz's Law: conductor moving to the right, giving rise to an induced current, which in turn causes a force to the left, opposing the motion.

Sometimes, even Chinese medical professionals don't believe this medical system. If you understand Faraday's Right Hand Law (Illustration Above), then you will know the electromagnetic field and the force are related that cannot be divided. And from that, the motor and generator then were developed – Question #15.

So, the human body structure is better than the automobile structure because the human body's battery or sphere field—Qi's loop system—seems (see previous Meridians illustrations) to have a wireless system and a magnetic field system besides the wire system or nerve system.

That's why it is hoped that the reader will go to practice Qi Gong first and then it will be easy to understand what is being described here.

The reason for those statements is that the Qi's loop system already contains an electrical system and a magnetic system, with functions that have similar points, as follows:

1....The Qi's flow is in only one direction, not reversible, although some people, after their learning moves to a higher level, can reverse the direction of flow—like AC, alternating current. (Why do the reversal? Any benefits? – Question #16)
Note: The benefits of reversal are many, including the fact that people can break through the location where Qi was blocked or a blood clot.

2....Qi can be divided into positive and negative (yang and yin). (Chinese philosophy, not proof? – Question #14)
Note: Since Qi's flowing has direction, then to give is yang (positive) and to receive is yin (negative).

3....Qi extends beyond our physical body. Some fish can send electric shocks to capture prey, and fireflies can flash a glow (that's also a chemical glow). Also, some humans can communicate with the spirit world and to tell people what is going to happen. All this is from the same source.

4....The directions of the earth's magnetic field and the sun's and moon's magnetic fields in combination will influence Qi's flow. (The full moon can affect some people.) That's why the practice of Qi Gong has rules to follow which depend on the timing and direction to face (east, south, etc.)

5....Animals may sense the earth's magnetic field. That's why migratory birds can fly south or north without missing their direction. But when thunder occurs, it will influence their direction. Sometimes, they may even lose their way.

6....When you practice Qi Gong, the more times your Qi's cycle flows, the more energy you accumulate. It's like taking a steel pin and rubbing it along the positive-negative alignment. The more times you rub the regular steel, the more magnetic force this regular still will get. This is why in people who have studied Qi Gong, the older they are, having practiced longer, the stronger will be their inner force. It's different from Western exercise such as boxing. When the boxer is over 30, his power is declining.

Note: Not only the energy you get more, but also the "Meridian" (the pathway of Qi) will be getting bigger, so that allows the bigger volume of "Qi" to pass through. Some "beginners" practice very hard, instead of the four hours of practice (maximum), and try to do 6 or even 8 hours. They hope to gain great results as soon as possible, but forget that the meridians are not growing that fast or big enough for a large volume of energy (Qi) to pass through. In the end, the person will be burned to death. This is the same as trying to use a small wire to let a large electrical current go through and that will cause a fire. The term of this trouble in Qi Gong is also called "getting fire" or "short."

7....Sphere field acupuncture points and all loops can be sensed but cannot be seen, just like magnetic force lines. However, when you check a few dead bodies, very often you will discover there is a swollen and hard tube appearing along the center line from the chest to below the navel. That's one part of the major loop system. It happens because Qi's flow stopped, so lots of body fluid stopped there and made it swollen.

8....Chinese medical books always say, "Blood is for carrying and Qi is for guarding or delivery." That means the blood is carrying nutrition and oxygen and waste products, but when blood goes from the heart through large arteries to veins to capillaries, then leaves and flows to the tissues, the force they depend on is not the heart any more, but Qi's force. Vice versa, from tissue, carrying back waste to veins also depends on Qi's force. This is the reason acupuncture or the use of pressure points can stop blood flow, and even make a person numb in a part of the body. There is no need to clamp the blood vessel—one needle or the pressure from a finger stops the flow. That was how China showed President Nixon: the Chinese doctors did surgery without anesthesia and less blood loss. Since then, acupuncture started to be legalized in the U.S. Some medical doctors who were licensed for acupuncture claimed that anesthesia by acupuncture is not true. It is because that what was taught in regular acupuncture school did not include the "Ear Acupuncture." The specialist in this is Dr. Li-Chun Hang in Florida.

From these few similar points and their special functions, it is obvious that Qi's function contains electrical and magnetic functions.

So the author thinks it is feasible to see the human body or an animal's body as a magnetic field and an electrical field combination.

Now, with this more comprehensive understanding of the human body structure according to the concepts herein described, it will be easier to discuss many problems, and AIDS is one of them.

CHAPTER 3

WHAT IS AIDS?

It is known that AIDS is Acquired Immune Deficiency Syndrome, which means that the immune system is damaged or destroyed and cannot defend itself from all kinds of germs and viruses, resulting in many kinds of illnesses. So, the major problem is the immune system deficiency.

But why is there this kind of disease?

A major reason is that the patient's body's magnetic field's force "Qi" declines very fast. In our human body, there is a natural immune force. It is a kind of acid-alkaline reaction and from that come the electric and magnetic function. Those produce the energy to let our cells have power to develop their immune function.

So only when the body's magnetic field has been or is being destroyed, the ability of the life power's production becomes weaker and weaker. That means it cannot supply enough energy efficiently to our immune cells so that they can fight the disease.

Moreover, it can even produce deformed cells or a virus during our tissue cells' regeneration metabolism and then make even more terrible damage.

In other words, even without an invasion by outside germs or viruses, this patient's body's life force is already getting weaker and weaker, and the cells in the tissues, the energy those cells can get becomes weaker, too.

All the tissue itself is then totally deformed and cannot absorb energy, which means it is getting closer to death because this whole body's tissue is being changed back to dust.

There is a spiritual dimension involved. This is the reason why many Qi Gong masters, when they reach a high level, can communicate with a spiritual field, especially the high-ranking monk or yoga master. They always look down on the human body as having no value because they all know that, after you removed the Qi from the human body, the rest is only dust.

So we may say that a major reason for AIDS is that the human body's electro-magnetic field is depleted, and the body is changing back to dust.

Some chapter questions (answers are provided later in this book):

Do we treat with drugs to kill the AIDS virus or skip the drugs? (Question #17)

AIDS drugs have been able to keep the disease under control and the patients now live longer because of the drugs.

What is the relationship between Qi Gong and drugs? (Question #18)

Are there certain herbs and foods that cooperate with Qi Gong? (Question #19)

CHAPTER 4

DEFINITION OF HOMOSEXUALITY

Generally, when we discuss the homosexuals' human rights, we tend to give too much attention to their love. We neglect or ignore their sexual practices or we're afraid to discuss them.

As a matter of fact, if the relationship of love and caring for each other did not result in a sexual relationship's existence, we would call them good friends instead of homosexual partners, so the real meaning of homosexual is a preference for homosexual intercourse.

The ways of intercourse such as (1) man and man, (2) woman and woman, (3) man and woman, (4) human and animal and all kinds of techniques are more than we can describe here.

Over all, we can summarize as follows:

1....Use of the man's organ in the woman's organ
2....Use of sexual toys or other implements
3....Use of the hand
4....Use of the man's organ in the partner's rectum
5....Use of the mouth or tongue to touch the sexual organs

1...Using male organ in female organ

This is generally the best, except both of them discharge body fluid and make the body a little weak. It's like taking the battery fluid out of the battery. That will make the battery's power decline. That's

31

why many athletes, a few days before the contest, or a paratrooper a day before jumping, if they have sexual intercourse, will become sub-normal easily and it will be easy for them to damage a leg or foot, from wasting the body fluid that protects the body. (Qi protect the body may not be the appropriate concept? – Qi is just like an air cushion in the joint.)

However, the male-female genital intercourse is best because the female receives the male's sperm fluid and also the male, after discharging the sperm fluid, absorbs the female's secretion. (Question #20: absorbing the female fluid is not accurate?– explained later in this book). In addition, this kind of intercourse is like putting two bar magnets' opposite poles together.

That is beneficial to both bodies and batteries.

That is why many young men or young women, before they have their first sexual experience always have a little problem. Most often, there is a little problem like pimples, but after normal sexual life it automatically recovers. This is what the Chinese say is Yin-Yang balance, or positive-negative balance. So it is important that human sexual intercourse actually should be matched to natural law and we can see it is good, with no harm to our body.

2…. Use of sexual toys or other implements

This is inferior to male-female intercourse because most of these are without magnetic force, and only facilitate discharge of body fluid. The person cannot receive the opposite sex's body fluid to balance the yin and yang. Nevertheless, roughly speaking, it is not too damaging.

However, if the lady puts the electrical toys in the vagina and plays very often, that will cause the magnetic influence and damage the magnetic field. So then, AIDS could happen too since the HIV virus could be produced, but different types from the homosexual men.

3….Masturbation

Generally, we mean that a hand seizes a penis, rubbing and pressing it so as to reach a climax and ejaculate the sperm. This depletes or damages the magnetic field, especially if a person does this very often. (Question: How can you prove there is damage? What is the damage?)

Answer: One indication of damage in self-masturbation is that when he raises his hand in the air, the hand will be shaking and he cannot hold it still, because the hand itself is the concentrated end of magnetic lines or force fields. The man's penis is also a very obvious magnetic concentrated point.

As a matter of fact, the human body's magnetic field, where it's concentrated, is just like the earth's. Besides the north and south magnetic poles, there are many magnetic points spread over the earth, such as the Bermuda Triangle and a locality in Wisconsin where people and trees stand at a slant, and other places. (Question #21: A better explanation or Internet links to explain such phenomena—explained later in this book. Some may consider these locations as fantasy of the imagination and not factual.)

Chinese doctors say the human body is a small cosmos. We can also say that the body is a small earth and the earth is a medium cosmos, and the electrons, atoms, and molecules are also micro-cosmos. Besides this, on the surface of the human body, the magnetic lines concentrate at points such as the (1) head, (2) genitals, (3) nipples, (4) tongue, (5) hand, (6) rectum, and so on. For details, if you would like to know more, please see the chart in Chapter 9. Then it will be easy to understand all of those major lines and what the loop is. (Question #22: Can you prove the magnetic lines exist? explained later in this book.)

4....Man and man or woman and woman

Now, we can figure out what the result will be when two same sex partners rub each other's magnetic points. After a short period of time of perhaps one to two months, the sphere field's or the battery's magnetic power to discharge energy will be weaker and weaker. (Question #23: This is a belief that cannot be measured? Explained later in this book.) That's why the energy cannot reach to the fingers or even the hand, which makes the hand tremble. Of course, that doesn't mean that all the people whose hands shake have the habit of masturbation. When some people are old or sick, their life power will be getting weak and they will have the same symptoms. (Question #24: Parkinson's disease is a neurological disease in the brain that can cause loss of control of the bodily movement. Nerve diseases are not considered? Explained later in this book.)

In other cases, some peoples' hands and feet always feel cold. That comes from the same reason—their energy is too weak or is blocked from flowing to the hands or feet. (Question #25: Blocked circulation will affect the hands and feet. Circulatory diseases are not considered, only magnetic explanation? Explained later in this book.)

From what we have discussed, about the most seriously damaging behavior to the body's magnetic field, is damage to the major cycle or loop, which occurs when men and men play with each other's magnetic points or when female and female do the same. (Question #26: If homosexual couples are successful over many decades, does that mean their magnetic fields have not been damaged? Explained later in this book.)

Damaging behavior includes using the hand or tongue, but the most damaging is that of using the penis in the rectum actively back and forth, because when two people are doing that, both of their Qi (life energy) are concentrating in the penis and rectum. (Question #27: What about any heterosexual couples who practice rectum intercourse, not just homosexuals? Are you saying that homosexuals cannot live long lives? Why is there a problem with the magnetism because the rectum is on the other side of the vagina area? Explained later in this book.)

When we review human history, homosexuality is not new. It is reported thousands of years ago in China that an emperor loved one of his ministers.

One day, after they had had rectal intercourse, the minister fell asleep and his body pressed the emperor's sleeves. Because the emperor loved the minister so much, he didn't want to wake him up, so he cut his own sleeves off and got up to work. That's the reason the Chinese call homosexuality the "cut-sleeve habit."

After a little period of time, this minister began looking very old very fast. The author believes he had developed what we now call AIDS. So, he was killed by the emperor for some false reason, because of the loss of his charm.

The Bible Story of Sodom

The author does not want to say the Bible is right or wrong and neither does he want to say the people were right or wrong. But as ancient information, it is very important to do the research.

Not only in China, but in Genesis 18:20 and 19:29, the destruction of the city of Sodom is described. The day when the angels came to Lot's house to warn him that God would rain fire to destroy the whole city, those two angels were seen by the men of the city and the men demanded that Lot send the angels outside to them. They even tried to break into Lot's house to get the two and rape them.

Lot begged them to leave his two guests alone and even said he would rather give his own two daughters instead, who were virgins, for their pleasure to try to change the situation. (That includes leaving his two daughters for them to have rectal intercourse.)

Now, the questions are: since Lot protected these two angels from rectal intercourse, he must know rectal intercourse is no good, but why? Why should Lot sacrifice his two daughters? (Is he a good man?) And if rectal intercourse is no good for angels, it must not be good for his daughters. What is the difference? Why was that behavior spurned by God?

From these questions, we can see a few conclusions: (1) rectal intercourse is no good for two angels (male or nonsexual), (2) but seems no harm for his two daughters, and (3) and men to men sex is spurned by God for some reasons. The author explained the Qi's Field was damaged and unclean, which not only would cause AIDS on the earth, but also polluted the souls of the people. So, they could not survive in Heaven just the same as people eat pork.

So, it can be said that the Sodom was spurned by God possibly because all the people had AIDS. The AIDS virus had already spread over the city. Otherwise, it would be absolutely impossible for any other "sin" to make a whole city be punished because God could not even find ten good men (those who didn't commit the sin). Later on, Jonah 4:10-11 records: "Then said the Lord, thou hast had pity on the gourd, for which thou hast not labored, neither madest it grow; which came up in a night, and perished in a night. And should not I spare Nineveh, that great city, where in are more than six thousand persons that cannot discern between their right hand and their left hand, and also much cattle?" (King James Version)

Here, the author found the "sin" should be changed to "unclean." That means their Qi Fields were damaged. And to keep "Qi" clean seems to involve the "holy" or so-called "superconductor"—this is the author's expression using a contemporary term.

Also, Matthew 10:11-15, Jesus told the disciples, "When you come to a town or village, go in and look for someone who is willing to welcome you, and stay with him until you leave that place. When you go into that house, say, 'Peace be with you.' If the people in that house welcome you, let your greeting of peace remain, but if they do not welcome you, then take back your greeting. And if some house or town will not welcome you or listen to you, then leave that place and shake the dust off your feet. I assure you that on the Judgment Day God will show more mercy to the people of Sodom and Gomorrah than to the people of that town."

From this paragraph, we can see that homosexual behavior is not that severe a sin as we have thought. But to burn the whole cities of Sodom and Gomorrah, the meaning seems to be to get rid of infectious diseases (such as AIDS or the black plague) more than to punish homosexual people. Of course, God had also wiped out humans during "Noah's flood."

Also, we can see the claim that "God loves homosexual people" seems right. But that does not mean gay men can be a pastor, just like "sacrificial animals" should not include pigs (pork).

In other words, God is holy. If people want to be with God, they should maintain themselves as clean as God. Otherwise, those people will be burned automatically. That explains: God insisted people should maintain themselves holy. Otherwise, they cannot get into Heaven. It is a surprise to say: "Satan is holy (clean)." That is why he could walk by in front of God and not be burned (John 1:6-7). And many good Christians will not be allowed into Heaven, because they are unclean. (Matthew 22:9-13). The guests from the street will be thrown back out to the street due to their being unclean.

Why are there so many people who would rather take part in anal intercourse instead of the vaginal intercourse? And why does it seem that they are addicted and cannot give it up?

Using the penis in the rectum is supposed to be the most comfortable, most exciting sexual behavior for the male because:

1...The anus is small, tighter than the female's vagina, and it is easier to control the tightening and loosening.

2....The diameter of the anus is about 1 to 2 inches; the vagina's opening can be about 2 to 3 inches.

3....All people naturally know how to use the anal sphincter to give pressure or to stop it, but very few women know how to use the vagina to give pressure. That's why, most of the time, when women go into delivery, they have to practice how to push before delivery. (Question #28: not sure if the delivery practice relates to vaginal intercourse—Explained later in this book.)

4....In the homosexual passive partner, the pressure upon the prostate during anal intercourse creates sexual excitation and the active partner, sometimes, prefers the tighter pressure of the anal sphincter muscle.

However, just as taking drugs, the practice of anal intercourse will make the person addicted, and will create a serious and terrible result which damages and destroys the health.

Now, let us temporarily put aside the relationship of anal intercourse to AIDS until later.

The damage to the rectum by anal intercourse already has been a big problem to which we have to pay attention.

When the author served in St. Mary's Immaculate Hospital in Queens, New York, he saw a few patients whose rectums had already become a big hole and could not close at all, with diameters of about 1½ inches.

In patients with the less serious problems, their rectums could not hold a rectal thermometer, and it was necessary to hold the thermometer in the rectum by hand to take the temperature.

In the more seriously damaged patients, bowel movement was already out of control and the feces came out little by little, so that their diapers had to be changed very often. When asked, they all said they were homosexuals.

Many doctors and nurses have seen this just as the author did.

The author recommends that no one should ever perform anal intercourse, because a person may become addicted and unable to quit. Also, a person can hurt his partner badly—but not himself.

CHAPTER 5

ETIOLOGY AND CONTAGION OF AIDS

In a previous chapter, we already mentioned how anal intercourse damages the human body's magnetic field, but what is the relationship to AIDS? Why are people who never do anal intercourse also affected, and why is it that even the infant cannot get rid of it?

Let's go for more detail and analyze it.

To begin with, because the same magnetic poles will repel each other, damaging each other's magnetic field, it is from this magnetic point (penis and anus), that damage to the body cells' magnetic field begins (each cell has its own magnetic field), which means that each cell has already changed its own nature.

We have learned that in the human body there are two kinds of cells. One is a permanent cell that doesn't metabolize and another that continues to regenerate, like skin.

In those tissues' cells that have the regeneration procedure, sometimes, because the magnetic fields of the cells themselves have been affected by some kind of change or influence, it would be very easy to get deformed cells—just like some change or influence during pregnancy can make it very easy to get deformed children—and, sometimes, even produce viruses.

For instance, like skin cancer, in which mostly the reason is too much sun, causing burns, we know in the sun's rays is a kind of light or radiation, and we know that the relationship between the light wave and electric wave and magnetic wave and force are four in one. That's why in the skin, if too much suntan is taken, regeneration will be influenced by the light and poison will be produced from the tissue and make for deformed cells. The cells start a rapid growth which is cancer.

And that kind of deformed cell will grow and spread; even though these visible cancer cells were cut off by surgery, it will continue to grow, if the etiology is not traced and cured. It will end up with the poison that will kill the patient.

In that case, the cancerous cells will affect the healthier skin cells, and we know these cancer cells did not come from outside, but were made by the patient's body itself.

When these deformed or materially-changed cells or the blood or the virus through the blood's circulation and magnetic circuit will change, the sphere field or battery's electrolyte will change the material inside the cells. It also will change this fluid's regenerative function and then how long can this battery or sphere field's function last?

Just like the automobile's battery—if it is connected the wrong way, it very often would burn down. Or, if a little of the electrolyte fluid from the burned-down battery were taken out and put into another good battery then defiantly the life of this good battery would be shortened too.

Now, since there are many different body fluids in the human body, including the man's semen, woman's secretion, saliva, blood, tears, and all kinds of fluids from various organs, and all kinds of body fluids always have these functions: (1) metabolism, (2) circulation, and (3) recycling—especially the man's semen and the woman's secretion. Sperm is possibly just the body's battery electrical fluid. (Question #29: Not so understandable why?—Explained later in this book.)

In an average man, the volume of semen in the body totals about 10 c.c. and the volume that can be replenished in one day is even more limited, unless he eats a dozen raw oysters which will help.

Then, if the semen is polluted, the symptom should show up very quickly. The timing should be shorter than if the blood were polluted or affected. (Question #30: The timing may not be a supported idea. Explained later in this book.)

However, how about the saliva? We all know the saliva itself is a very important secretion. Also, there is a close relationship between the saliva and the semen. (Question #31: close?) They seem to be correlated in volume and imply to each other. That's why when you sit down doing the "leading Qi exercise" the saliva will be secreted automatically which, in Chinese medical books we call "golden sauce" or "jade fluid;" and after sexual intercourse is completed, right away you will feel very thirsty. (Question #32: possibly thirsty from heavy breathing that dried up the saliva? Explained later in this book.)

Likewise, if you spit out clean saliva repeatedly, you will feel tired right away. (Question #33: tired?) For the same reasons, in the people who have AIDS, the saliva will be secreted less and less; the semen secretion is also less and less. In other words, the body's battery fluid is declining. That's why its life force or power is getting weaker and weaker. So that, in all kinds of parts like the organs or tissues of the body, the energy or magnetic force available will be to the same degree less and less.

Then the skin will become drier and drier and older. Normally skin is smooth, flexible, bright with light, and firm. On the contrary, when a person has AIDS, the skin is dark, old, dry, and loose with wrinkles.

Also, we can figure that those tissues within the body probably have a similar situation—shrunk, old, without power inside.

Finally, when all the electrical fluid is affected, when there is no new or normal fluid replenished at all and the old fluid is totally changed or the new fluids are also changed (deformed), that is the time the man is really dying. So the Chinese doctor calls the man dead, says that the candle wick is dried out and all the tallow (wax) is gone. (Question #35)

This kind of symptom is evident in the difference between an infant and an old man who is dying. We can see that the baby's whole body is very round, but that doesn't mean the body is full of fat, only that the magnetic power is very full, just like a brand new battery. In Chinese, we describe that as full of Qi, like a balloon; we say someone is an old man when he is short of Qi or life force, so his skin is drying out and without the brightness and pink color of a young healthy person.

With the saliva's pollution, the result should be very serious too, but because the saliva, after being polluted through a kiss or oral sex, won't be absorbed by the mouth into the salivary glands (these glands secrete, not absorb) and because it still has to go through the digestive system. Contaminated saliva has to get through a lot of digestive fluid which has a strong ability to kill germs or virus in the saliva, so after the polluted is assimilated into the blood, the possibility of danger is already declined.

One reason is that the AIDS virus needs a living environment the same as our body's cells, and must be in the tissue of the body. In the system of digestion, although it's in our body, actually it is outside of the tissue's living environment. That's why, when the saliva is polluted, its effect is much lower; it almost can be ignored. However, if the polluted saliva is directly injected into the Qi channel or blood vessel, the trouble could be very serious, as in cunnilingus, but not in fellatio.

The other body fluids' influence we can figure out from this. So we can judge that the effect through the blood or sexual intercourse must be direct and not interrupted because the virus and our body cells or blood are very compatible and do not expel each other.

The virus will be very easily carried to the tissue and sphere field and then grow more widespread, then damage more blood and more cells' magnetic field.

Now, let's go back to the etiology of AIDS. After we recognize there are the magnetic field and battery in our body, we will know that the syndrome is not really horrible because it's only the result. What we should be concerned about is its cause—the immune system deficiency. In other words, that's caused by the body's battery's damage. The AIDS initial cause can be summarized as follows:

1....The sphere field's (body's battery) being totally burned down. This is the most serious damage. Just like putting a car battery's positive and negative together, it will soon be burned down and cannot be re-charged.

This symptom almost cannot be seen in the human body because the sphere field in the body appears only to function with magnetic force and not electrical force. We can see only the symptom of the magnetic force declining, but cannot see the symptom of burn-down, except those people have the special ability to give electrical shock or the people who have learned high-level Qi Gong. After the sphere field is burned down, the person will be dead.

2....Frequent anal intercourse makes the sphere field's magnetic power decline. Although we say frequent, actually we don't have the real data, but once a week could qualify to be frequent because generally after intercourse a person needs 24 hours to recover. After anal intercourse, because the magnetic power is declining, a person needs two to three times the amount of time to recover. In general, intercourse between healthy people, although the man's semen can recover to original volume (actually only 80% to 90%) within one day, the energy in the tissue already has one day's depletion. Therefore, one would need 48 hours to refuel all depletions. Then, if multiplied by three, this is equal to six days. Therefore, once in six days can be regarded as frequent.

Moreover, when doing anal intercourse, the person receiving will be hurt more seriously than the one giving. Those who have learned Qi Gong will understand that when doing anal intercourse the rectal muscle will be expanded and contracted, and then the Qi's flow or magnetic force will send magnetic waves which will have a destructive effect on the receiver's magnetic or Qi loop. The one who is doing the giving is only giving out Qi and not receiving it, so the flow is only in one direction. The one who receives, because of contact directly with the major loop of both, will have the same magnetic flow as putting the same ends of two magnets together—positive/positive or negative/negative.

With male-female anal intercourse, if the female receives, she may be less injured because women are considerably different from men and it would, therefore, be almost the same as vaginal intercourse as far as the magnetic loop is concerned. However, it still would do her damage, such as injury to the rectum. (Women catch AIDS too in various ways. —Explained later in this book – Question #36.)

When there are two positives together, it demagnetizes the receiver and that countervails the magnetic power from the sphere field, making it weaker and weaker, and thus the immune system weaker and weaker too.

When the immune system's strength declines to a certain level, all kinds of germs and viruses can invade or attack the body. Usually the immune system can defend the body with no problem, but now comes the syndrome called AIDS.

3....As described in (2), not only is the immune system's ability getting weaker, but all the body's tissue cells and blood metabolism ability also get in trouble. When their magnetic fields are damaged or destroyed, then they will produce deformed cells or blood or poison virus. So far the medical industry knows there are many different kinds of AIDS viruses. Suppose these kinds of viruses are created from our body, not introduced from outside, unless from another person, but overall, still created from the human body. Also, different tissues will create a different virus under different levels of magnetic field damage.

4....All these deformed cells or viruses of course will be like normal cells with the ability to multiply and make more trouble.

5....The other healthy people, or the infant, will get this virus through heredity, from damaged genes or through damaged blood from the mother.

6….From the above description, we may infer that the AIDS virus must have its own living circumstances. These include temperature, magnetic field, nutrition, and oxygen level within. We may consider the semen, the blood and the woman's secretion as especially good environments.

On the other hand, the ocean's water is not a good environment for the AIDS virus, so the ocean water cannot be polluted by the virus unless by coincidence the virus gets into the fish's blood or the blood of a human in the water before the virus dies.

Therefore, if the oceans can clean it out, then for the Long Island beaches, when hypodermic needles wash ashore, we shouldn't be afraid of the AIDS disease being spread in water, but we should still be careful of the needles because perhaps there are still some viruses in the needle.

CHAPTER 6

HOW TO PREVENT AIDS CONTAGION

So far, lots of advertisements insist that the condom will prevent AIDS infection or contagion. Here it must be emphasized very seriously that the condom is not safe.

That's right. In a certain way, it will prevent the pollution of the body fluid. However, THE CONDOM WILL NOT PREVENT DAMAGE TO THE MAGNETIC FIELD CAUSED BY ANAL INTERCOURSE.

For example, you may take two pieces of magnetic steel—one in a condom and the other placed on a table. Then observe them and see whether they still have the relationship of repelling or attracting as magnets. As you will see, the rubber condom absolutely cannot prevent the magnetic power's influence. So even when two males use the condom to have anal intercourse, when the penis is rubbing in the colon, the resulting damage to the magnetic field is the same.

For another example, all humans, animals and plants are like pieces of needles. When a powerful steel magnet rubs on the small needle, the needle will get magnetized and become a magnetic needle, which we'll call needle (a). Then we pick another piece of a regular needle and call it (b), to rub with needle (a) or even just put them together. So, needle (b) will be magnetized. However, the original needle (a)'s magnetic power will decline. If we use this needle (a) to work with more regular needles, eventually needle (a)'s magnetic power will totally disappear. However, to the permanent magnetic steel, this will not happen.

This is why the ancient Chinese used to say it's all right for the infant to be held by senior people once in a while, but don't let the infant sleep with senior people, because the senior person's body will automatically drain the infant's Qi (body energy). That will make the senior people live longer, but the infant will decline and, although he grows up, he will not live as long. (People who don't believe in body magnetism will want statistical evidence of this – Question #37.)

A similar story happened in the Bible in I Kings 1:1-4. King David had a young girl, Abishag, sleep with him when he was old.

Let me bring another example: we know in the Bible, there are many types of miracles to cure people from death. But one example is very special and interesting: II Kings 4:32: When Elijah arrived, he went alone into the room and saw the boy lying dead on the bed. He closed the door and prayed to the Lord. Then he lay down on the boy, placing his mouth, eyes, and hands on the boy's mouth, eyes, and hands. As he laid stretched out over the boy, the boy's body started to get warm. Elijah got up, walked around the room, and then went back and again stretched himself over the boy. The boy sneezed seven times and then opened his eyes.

This procedure, as a matter of fact, is "Qi Gong healing." He could just do as Jesus did when he ordered the child to wake up and get out of bed.

Here the author has emphasized that he has found the Bible is not fiction. As a matter of fact, when he reads and studies it, many things just coincidental can be matched with the Chinese ancient book that said, and with scientific reasons. So, please don't just ignore it, but you may question the author for a reasonable answer.

So, we can conclude theoretically, if healthy people hug the AIDS patients or the old man who is dying or even if man and man or woman and woman hug each other, both persons' magnetic power will decline, unless they hug in a certain way.

On the other hand, there are some ways to heal or cure dead people from drowning or hanging or freezing (See methods later in this book entitled "Death Caused by Hanging or Strangling"), provided that it is done within 24 hours or if the heart is still a little warm, even though it stopped beating is to let another living person make full length body contact and use that person's magnetic power to stimulate the "dead" person's life power. It always works. (Question #38: The heart would be cold before 24 hours. Do the Chinese practice this today? Why don't the Chinese doctors tell the world? It seems like a big secret. –Explained later in this book.)

However, we don't need to make much of a trifle either, because in the body automatically there are the regenerative and healing functions so that when minor damage occurs, the body supposedly can conquer it and recover by itself. That's like when we are using a new car's battery to charge a junk car's weak battery, the good battery itself will get a little damage more or less, but because the good car's engine is running it won't get hurt much. Nevertheless, if we continue to charge many weak batteries, eventually the new battery will be damaged too.

This description is to illustrate that the people's general idea about the condom's being able to prevent AIDS is not complete and a little mistaken, although the other general idea is still correct.

Now, we just summarize as follows:

1....Absolutely avoid the behavior of anal intercourse, even with a condom, as that still cannot prevent damage to the body's magnetic field, and with it, the immune system.

2....If making love with people you don't know, it is better to use the condom to avoid the body's fluid's pollution.

3...People of the same sex must avoid using the tongue on one another's genitals, as this behavior will result in destroying the magnetic field, and its damage level is nearly that of anal intercourse.

4....Avoid masturbation (Question #39: needs further explanation as a reminder).

CHAPTER 7

HOW TO CURE (HEAL) AIDS

If we want to heal the AIDS syndrome, first we have to heal the auto immune deficiency.

When the immune system's ability to heal is deficient, basically it's because the sphere field's power is not strong enough, no matter whether it is caused by using up too much energy or caused by magnetic field destruction. The deficiency of the immune system then allows many diseases to happen.

If we don't heal the base first, we will just waste time and money. There are many strange diseases that modern medicine cannot solve, like cancer and AIDS. They all have the same characteristics:

1…No one knows where the disease came from. (We know some causes of cancer. Example, skin cancer caused by too much exposure to the sun – Question #40.)

2…It cannot be healed by antibiotics. (radiation and chemo therapies can work on some cancers – Question #41.)

3…The living conditions of all viruses are unknown to such an extent that it is difficult to create or synthesize a sample.

These problems occur because scientists neglect the influence of the body's magnetic field.

So the author appeals to all scientists to start work right away, starting with learning Qi Gong, to discover the relationship between the living being and its magnetic field; then, from that, find or develop the medicine or the way which can help restore the function of the body's sphere field as well as the medicine or the way to destroy the virus.

Of course, before the new medicine or new way can be discovered, we have to use what we know now and apply that right away.

According to what we know so far, we can focus on the idea of healing the damaged magnetic field. So far, the only ways we have found to focus on the magnetic field theory which we can use are Chinese herb medicine, Qi Gong and acupuncture. (Drugs now exist that extend the lives of AIDS patients – Question #42)

Actually, in many patients who have the disease and thought to be incurable in western systems, after they learn Qi Gong the situation mostly improves, especially after they practice it for five years. Mostly, they can completely recover.

Of course, there is no data to prove this. But, if people go to the Internet to check "Fa Lung Da Far"—the most well-developed division of "Qi Gong" during the past thirty years, people will find some kind of evidence—through their witness.

When starting all the herb medicines or acupuncture, they serve these functions:

I…..Replenish the sphere field's energy.
II….Recover the sphere field's magnetic function to normal.
III…Change the interior forms of the tissues' magnetic fields.
IV…Replenish the energy in the tissues.

Many tissues become mutants, sometimes not because the energy in the sphere field is not enough but just like in acupuncture anesthesia, when the energy of the sphere field, while it has been transferring to the tissue, is blocked or interrupted, so the energy can't supply the tissue.

So the way to solve it is to focus on this kind of situation to clear the paths for the energy to flow. In this kind of case, the best instance is lupus patients or people with stroke.

In Chinese martial arts, there is a special way to fight, called "strike at the vital point." It is just like in acupuncture, to press a special vital point so that the opponent's body or hand or leg or organ cannot function; there is also a special way to resolve it, to make the numb parts recover the sense again. All this is the same theory. And typical examples in sickness and their treatment are Alzheimer's and multiple sclerosis.

If we want to heal or cure this kind of disease which could not be cured by antibiotics, one of these that is especially representative is AIDS, which must be cured starting from energy's replenishment.

As to the tissues and the sphere field and all the procedures, we can summarize as follows:

I…Replenish the energy of the sphere field. We have many ways to do that:

A…Light/mild exercise

Exercise both mornings and evenings, but not at noon: Jogging, walking, climbing, also slowly doing gymnastics or performing Tai Chi Chuan. Absolutely, never over-exercise—not too heavy, just work or act until slightly perspiring, but not breathless or panting. Don't overburden or stress the heart; then the exercise is acceptable.

This is like an automobile stored in a garage. We have to start the engine at least once a week or after a couple of months the battery's energy will be all gone. However, if we drive the car for racing, then it will hurt the engine. So, over-exercise is not good for the patient.

B…Replenish by eating

Eat more food which is good for replenishing Qi, such as milk, beef, eggs, and honey, and don't eat non-kosher foods such as pork, shrimp, crab (shellfish) or fish without scales, nor scallion, garlic, onion, hot chili, hot pepper, at least until you recover. The so-called non-kosher food will either block the production of the human body's magnetic energy or will easily promote sexual desire and waste the body fluid or semen, and will deplete the energy of the sphere field.

From this, we can figure out that the kosher food of the Hebrews by theory is because God wants the human being close to Him, not far away from Him, and this non-kosher food will make the body fluid impure or polluted, or make waste the body fluid through sexual contact because that will stimulate the sexual appetite.

Actually there is a relationship which cannot be divided between the human spirit and the Qi, energy in the sphere field. That's why generally speaking, in the monk or priest or nun, the spiritual level is higher than in other people, especially after learning Qi Gong up to the higher level. Then you will sense the information is flowing in the spiritual field as the person is becoming clairvoyant or like a prophet.

In the book which teaches how to practice Qi Gong, there are the same kinds of regulations about food as found in the Bible in Leviticus Chapter 11 that teaches about kosher and non-kosher foods, including not eating ice. If we trace to the reason for these regulations, we will figure out that they come from those people who reach to the higher levels of Qi Gong, because they can sense when they eat it, what is good and what is bad for the human body. Then they wrote down those experiences and gave them to the later generations.

The most representative of these is an ancient Chinese emperor Wonder Farmer, who left a book entitled *Wonder Farmer's Hundreds of Herbs* that is so rich in knowledge about all kinds of plants that, even after a thousand years, now our modern western medicine is not as rich as this. All the prescriptions of the Chinese doctors are still based on it. It is generally believed that this book is not a collection by many Chinese doctors, but really comes from this one Wonder Farmer.

(The author wonders if he is the elder son of Adam—Cain identified in the Bible as a farmer, because ancestors of the Chinese is a woman called female Va; she is very beautiful. Also, she seemed to regret what she did as a big mistake and tried to make it up. So, mother and son came to China. And Cain's (son) was given a special ability (Genesis 4:15): "So, the Lord put a mark on Cain to warn anyone who met him not to kill him.")

For example, only from one in ancient times could tell the difference about:

a.. Rhinoceros horn

Western doctors said Chinese thought their function is like Viagra and for that to kill a rhinoceros is not good. Did they study? No. And just to protect the rare animal, prohibit the killing of the animal and selling their horns is not right.

The real truth in the book of *Wonder Farmer's Hundred of Herbs*: The function of powder from the horn is to resolve the high fever (such as lupus) and the toxin from the fever. It has nothing to do with sex at all.

To use: the horn of the male only. No the female's. (Its medical function is weak.) The horn located at the forehead is good. Not from the nose.

To acquire: The horn will fall off like a nail each year. After it falls off, the rhinoceros would usually bury the fallen off part in the ground. So, the people need to take it must hide and watch.

Quality: Separate according to the print on the horn. A print that is bigger is better than one that is fine and delicate. A flower print is better than a dark, black one.

Command: Even in the 21st century, does anyone do this research? No. Why not simply study the book which the author has studied? Then why did they prohibit to use it as medicine so arbitrarily?

b.. Gingko

Western doctors of western companies emphasized that gingko is good for memory and they made lots of money. Later on, some people claimed that it is not good for the female's period. And it seems it had toxins. So, some doctors just said that herbs are no good.

The real truth is in the *Wonder Farmer's Hundreds of Herbs*: The function of gingko: (1) warm up the lungs, (2) relieve coughing and panting, (3) reduce urine, (4) kill bacteria or small worms, and (5) reduce phlegm. It has nothing to do with memory.

To use: usual dose around 15-20 grams. If one takes one thousand pieces at one time (roughly taking that as a meal), people will die, because of Qi's clogging.

If the person eats Gingko with eels, that will cause a loss of strength in the legs.

From these two examples, people can easily tell the difference: who is lying? Who did the study? Who did research? Who had the better solution?

Doctors look down on the Chinese herbs—and considered them unscientific. Actually people were cheated by western doctors who said rhino horn is for sex, gingko is for the brain, totally without scientific evidence. They blamed the Chinese herbs after they were found not true.

C. Take Medicine to Replenish Energy

Get advice from a good Chinese doctor and get prescriptions to replenish energy, such as ginseng or compound herbs. However, do not take on your own without a doctor's direction, because if you take too much or take it in an incorrect way, it will have a side-effect. It's like when you charge a battery the voltage should not be too strong or too weak.

Ginseng in the Chinese medical book is called the king of medicines. Yet, so far, the western specialists cannot find its functions. The major reason is the Chinese doctors all know that ginseng is very good to help replenish Qi. In this book, the author calls it magnetism, which is a western concept. Also, it will help to stop wasting Qi. Sometimes, in childbirth, bleeding cannot be stopped. Chinese doctors always give ginseng to women so this may be the reason why. They are told to hold it in the mouth, so the blood will stop.

Another example is: if breast feeding mothers eat ginseng, the milk flow will diminish or even stop. From this, we can see how ginseng protects humans' Qi. Again, when people make ginseng tea or herbal portions containing ginseng, there is always a prohibition: never use a metal wok or pot. Always use china or pottery. The reason, the author thinks is that the metal has the function of eliminating magnetism or Qi, and reduces the effect of medicine.

Another prohibition during the period of taking ginseng is to never eat any peanuts because ginseng and peanuts are destructive to each other. If people take ginseng using a wrong method or too much, they will have the phenomenon of hypertension and tinnitus. The author thinks from what the above specialists should be able to find what the ginseng's real function is and get more knowledge about Qi. Therefore, to find a good doctor is very important to get the right prescription, otherwise, no matter how much money and time has been spent, it is in vain.

And so it is to be hoped that in the near future, modern scientists will develop new medicines, the functions of which would be to increase or decrease the magnetic power (Qi) in the sphere field. Then medical treatment can be more nearly complete.

D..Acupuncture: Asking the Acupuncturist to Cure

The acupuncturist doctor must be well informed about the acupuncture technique intended to increase or replenish magnetic energy (Qi), and to release magnetic energy.

Actually, these kinds of special techniques are developed from Qi Gong, and experts have found out that all those acupuncture points on the body, just like switches in an electrical system, not only can be turned on and off (acupuncture's local anesthetic), but also can be charged or discharged; so they can be used to increase or stimulate the function and the secretion of all kinds of organs. These principles also can be used to release magnetic energy which is excessively accumulated in some places, like rectifiers or transformers. It is also appropriate to note that manual acupuncture is required; the machine needle acupuncture method currently popular is not effective for this kind of special treatment. (How can you prove what you say? –Explained later in the book – Question #43.)

E.. Learning Qi Gong (or Yo-Ga)

So far, this is the easiest, most direct and most efficient way. This method has had more than two thousand years' application in China, India, Japan and other countries. Also, the expense involved in learning, compared to today's medical expense, is much less. The cost can be estimated at between 500 and 2,000 U.S. dollars for three months, which should be an adequate period. After three months, one already can practice the techniques by oneself at home, checking back with the teacher occasionally. Unfortunately, the oriental medical system is infiltrated with charlatans, but with Qi Gong, the student usually can see the result within one month's practice, and classmates' improvements are also obvious.

Of course, to learn Qi Gong, one must look for a good teacher. A good teacher not only can instruct in an efficient manner, but will advise the student of possible adverse reactions along the way. A good teacher will constantly correct the student physically as well as educationally so that problems do not develop. Working with a teacher is essential for best results. An effort to economize by self-instruction from books or tapes would be self-defeating, since one-on-one guidance is invaluable.

F.. Mechanically Charged Method

The author believes that after acknowledging and proving the relationships between the human body and electromagnetic and magnetic fields, scientists must be able to develop a kind of new machine which can charge the power (magnetic energy or Qi) into the sphere field or directly into the tissue. Such a machine would be effective even if people exhaust their energy, such as in excessive sexual activity or in the effects of aging or a lengthy illness. In the case of AIDS patients, their battery (sphere field) has been damaged. Also, the semen has been contaminated, as long as it is not 80%-100%, after recharging several times, the battery function should gradually return to normal. We say "gradually," because this kind of recharge cannot be done all at once. In cases of being totally burned down, we must charge a little bit, then wait for spontaneous healing include the volume and quality of the semen by the body itself. Little by little, the battery recovers a bit, then can stand to be more charged, then can produce (or provide) more energy. These are cause and result of each other. That's why even after you have learned Qi Gong, it is still necessary to take at least about three years to recover completely.

We know lots of so-called "death," but as long as the body's battery (sphere field) is not burned out completely, there must be some way to recharge it, and then the body can be revived. There is indication of this in phenomena in which people have dies for various reasons (usually some organ stops working but is not totally damaged), the doctor says the brain waves and heartbeat are stopped; but during delivery to the morgue or even the graveyard, sometimes, a person will come to life again, and remain alive for years more. This is because the battery's (sphere field's) function is working again, so that the malfunctioning organ revives. This is the same as the car that can't start because the power doesn't go through, but you can hold the positive wire, shake it, and, sometimes, start the car.

Another example: many a "dead" body has been put into a box and buried, then, after a few years, exhumed; on checking the body, often it will be found that the body's hair and nails have grown for about a year after being buried. (The time length may be incorrect – Explained later in the book.) That means this dead person was not really dead when he was buried, because his battery still supplied energy that made the hair and nails continue to grow. This kind of phenomenon is unlikely, however, with persons who have died of

AIDS because their batteries are totally burned out and cannot supply any more energy.

It must again be emphasized: the real definition of "death" should be that the battery (sphere field) is completely burned out.

G...Pray

This method is easy to say, yet difficult to do properly, First of all, you have to trust in God. Secondly, you have to depend on God one-hundred percent. Any doubt will make your prayer ineffective. For example, in Matthew 14:25-31: It is between three and six o'clock in the morning. Jesus came to the disciples walking on water. When they saw him walking on water, they were terrified. "It is a ghost," they said, and screamed with fear. Jesus spoke to them at once, "Courage." he said. "It is I. Don't be afraid." Then Peter spoke up. "Lord, if it is really you, order me to come out on the water to you." "Come," answered Jesus. So, Peter got out of the boat and started walking on the water to Jesus. But when he noticed the strong wind, he was afraid and started to sink down in the water. "Save me, Lord." he cried. At once, Jesus reached out and grabbed hold of him and said, "What little faith you have. Why did you doubt?" Because God could create human beings from dust, He should be able to save people from changing back to dust. Therefore, the author has to mention it here. And in the divisions of Christians, he found the division "Church of True Jesus." Their prayers are very powerful. (The author belongs to the Reform Church.) But because when they are praying, most of the people are jumping automatically like crazy. So, this division is not that popular. However, any believer, as long as he ever jumped, he will never leave his trust anymore, no matter what the scientist said, because he knew the Holy Spirit is with him.

II...Changing the sphere field's magnetic function: Recover the sphere field's magnetic function so that it returns to normal.

Because in an old battery, if the fluid contains too many impurities or if there is a wrong connection so that the sulfuric acid is not so good as new fluid, or if the electrode has been burned down so that the power is getting very weak. Still, after being recharged, the battery can be used for a little while. The difference is that the sphere field is better than a battery because the sphere field can spontaneously cure itself after being recharged and can then gradually become "new" again. So we can say that I and II are two in one. When we replenish the magnetic power in the sphere field, the magnetic power is already changing the function of the sphere field during the process. Up to now, the author was always wondering: Is it possible for doctors to change the AIDS patients' semen with a healthy person's semen, just like changing the blood? That would perhaps have a good outcome immediately.

To facilitate the flow of magnetic power in the Qi pathways (including the blood vessels, tendons, nerves and bones) or break through the blocked positions in these pathways: all these techniques in Qi Gong we call, "Breaking through the Pulse Vascular." (Questions & Answers – Question #45)

After a person learns until he can feel a mass of hot energy accumulating in his sphere field, and can sense this energy running back and forth in his body, it is time for the Qi Gong teacher to teach him how to use his mind to control this Qi sphere moving in his body. Under the teacher's instruction, the Qi sphere will follow the student's will, section by section, to open a connecting road or to remove the block in the Qi's passage (pulse vascular). It is the same as using running water to wash away the silt which blocks or chokes a sewer; gradually the pulse vascular may be gotten through the Qi-sphere. This kind of phenomenon happening in people who are over 30 years of age will be more difficult, because the silt is generally more than in young people's pulse vascular, especially in the tendons and the bones. That's why people over 30 years usually feel their muscle is no longer as flexible as when they were younger, and when they are over 40 years, even the bones are becoming fragile and brittle.

When sick people try to break through the pulse vascular, they will find resistance in unhealthy areas. For instance, if a person's leg is paralytic, either he needs to take time to move the Qi-sphere through the meridians to his feet and then back or he may move the Qi-sphere back and forth outside the leg, but in line of vessels just like the magnetic line. However, the energy can go through inside only a little. (See illustrations of 12 Meridians and 8 Vessels)

Illustrations also in Chapter 2

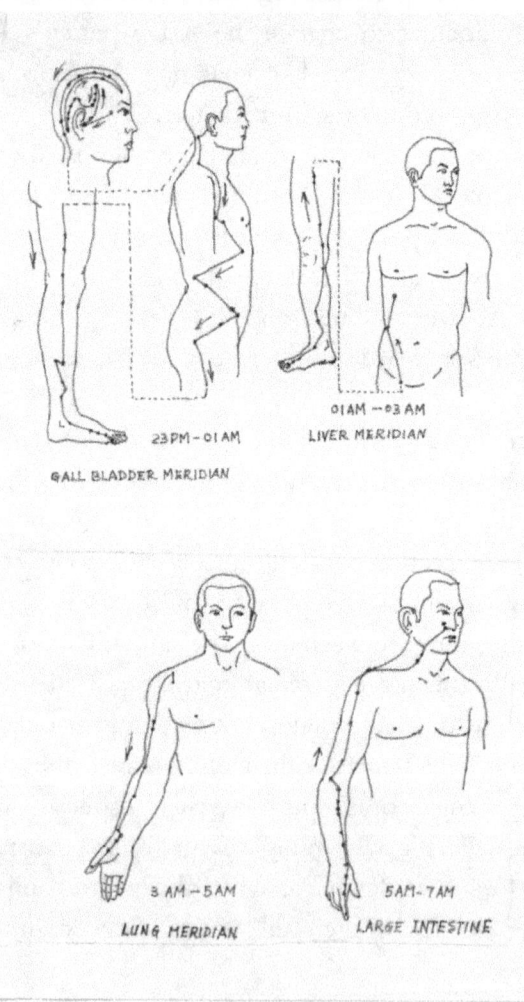

23 PM - 01 AM
GALL BLADDER MERIDIAN

01 AM - 03 AM
LIVER MERIDIAN

3 AM - 5 AM
LUNG MERIDIAN

5 AM - 7 AM
LARGE INTESTINE

Figure 1A

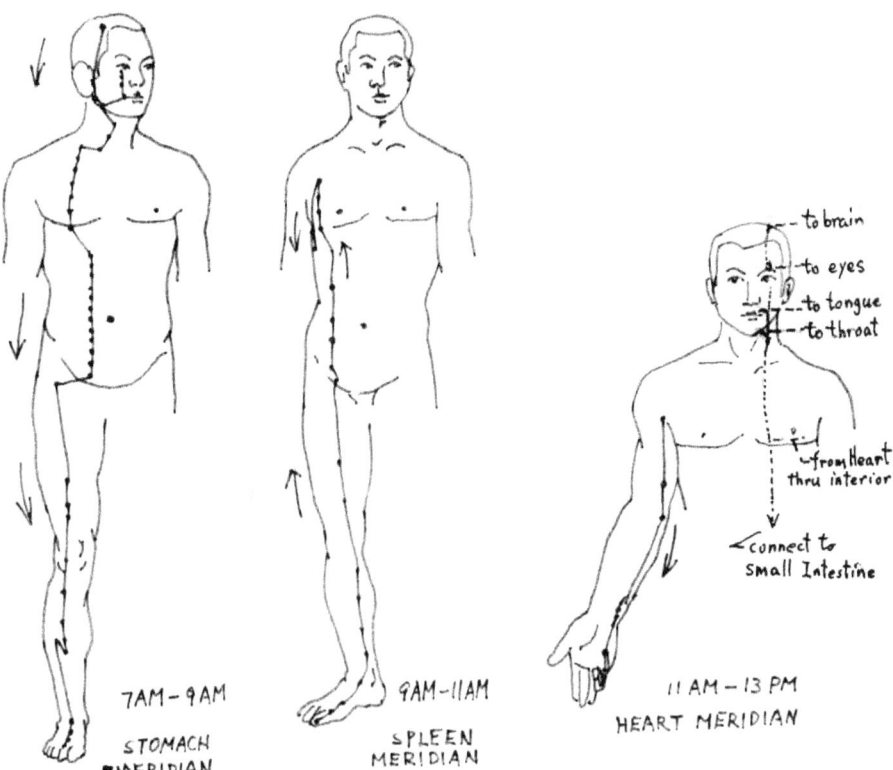

Figure 2B

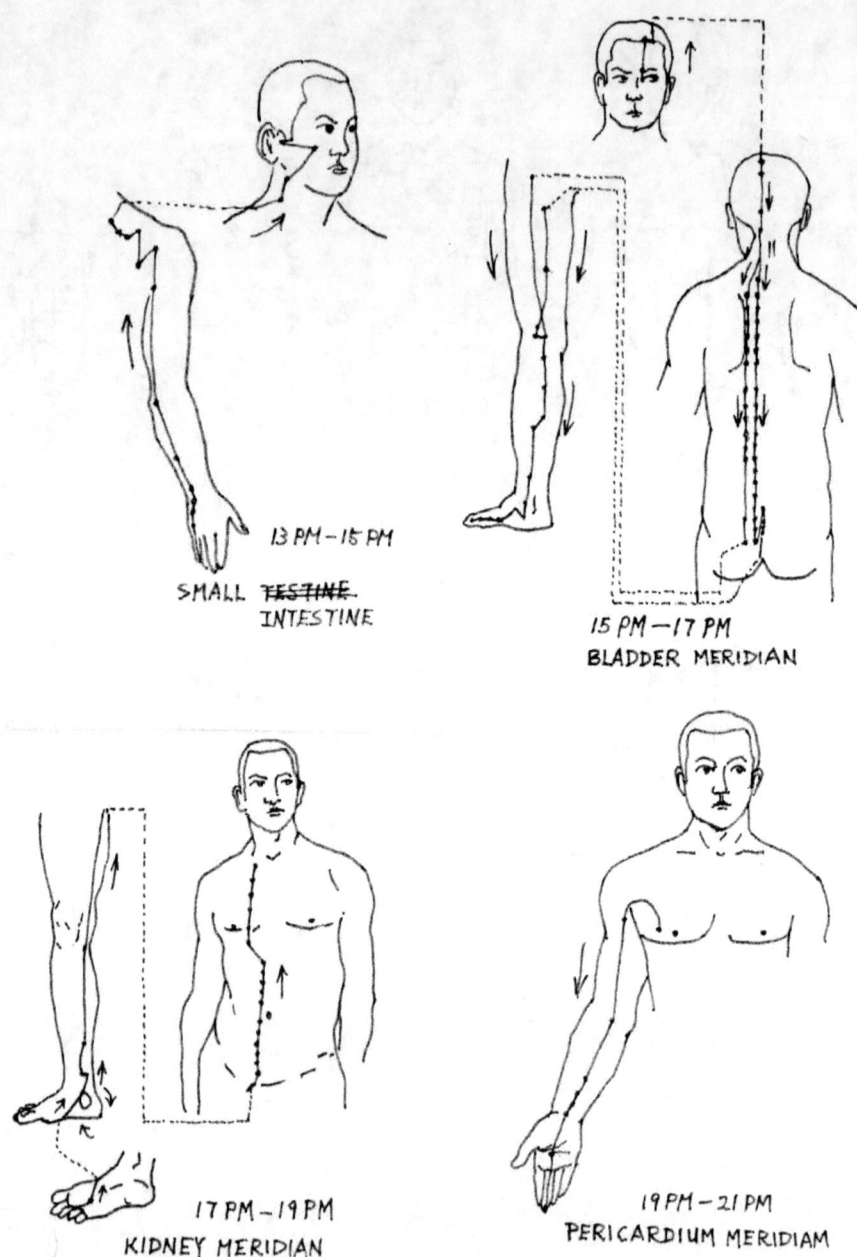

13 PM – 15 PM
SMALL ~~TESTINE~~ INTESTINE

15 PM – 17 PM
BLADDER MERIDIAN

17 PM – 19 PM
KIDNEY MERIDIAN

19 PM – 21 PM
PERICARDIUM MERIDIAM

Figure 3C

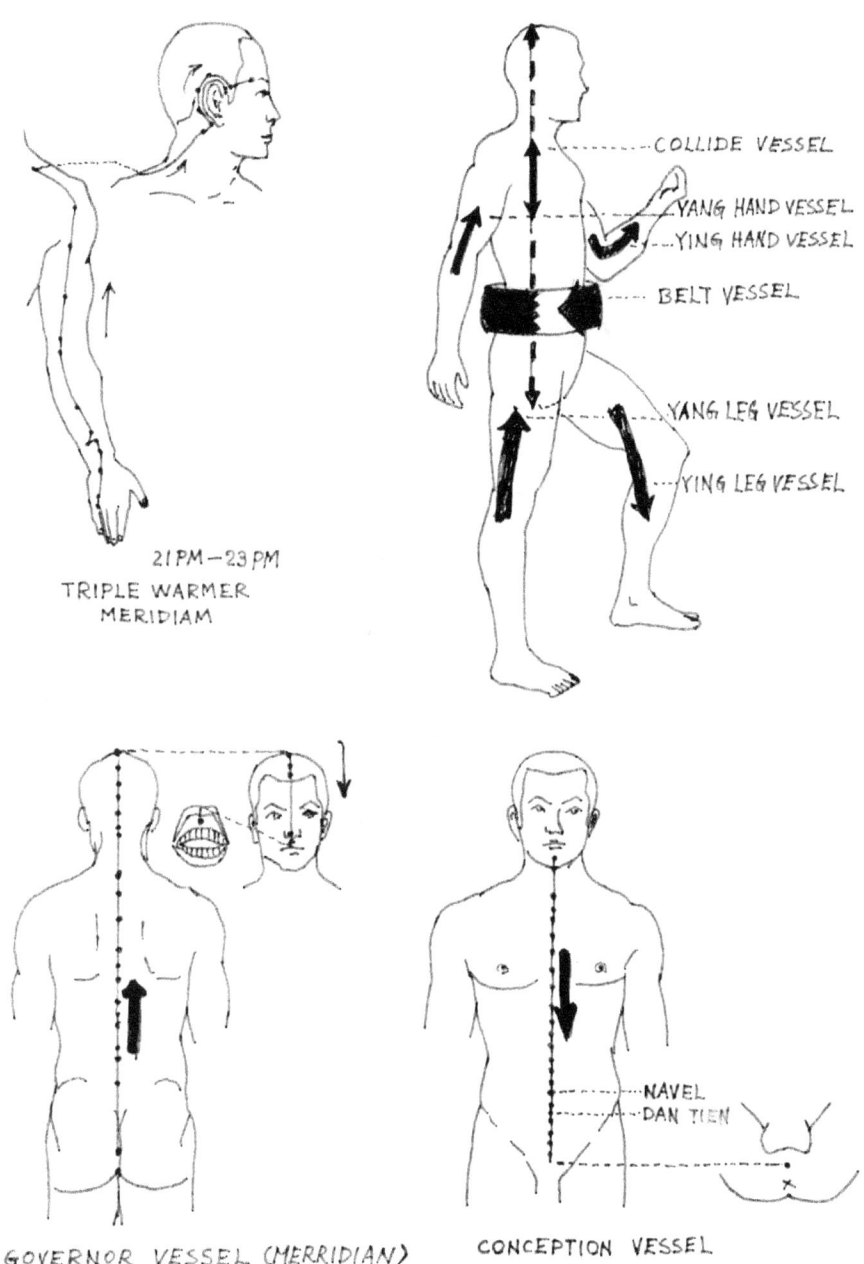

Figure 4D

So, after a person learns Qi Gong to a high level, he will recover from fatigue very fast, because all his vascular energy over his whole body is flowing freely with the Qi-sphere. In other words, the electric resistance changes to very low, and becomes a superconductor, so that the energy's delivery is very fast and volume very large; also the acid matter which makes people tired will be eliminated faster than in ordinary people, so he can shorten his sleeping time, like the great monk, Hai Den (Sea Lits), who didn't even need to sleep, only sat cross-legged for about three to four hours a day to generate his own energy.

III. Change the magnetic function in mutated tissues or organs

When a person has the ability to break through the pulse vascular, he can move the Qi-sphere to any mutated tissue or sick organ such as the heart, liver, lung, kidney, spleen, pancreas, and uterus—anywhere in the body. When the Qi-sphere moves through organs, it will automatically improve their function. Generally speaking, if a person can keep on moving the Qi-sphere to heal the sick or mutated tissue or organ for one week, he will stop it from getting worse; curing it completely may need one to three years.

IV. Replenish energy in tissue or organs

As in III, during the curing process, they will get energy gradually so that their functions will return to normal and produce their marked effect completely.

It is appropriate to note that one cannot see the vascular of Qi, but can only sense it, even though the routes of Qi's passing are just like blood vessels, containing aorta, arteries, veins and capillaries. Moreover, they go through skin, hair, nails, blood, muscle, and bones. In other words, Qi runs through all of the body, making the body's every part alive and growing.

We know every living person has Qi, and to learn Qi is to learn how to generate Qi, to accumulate it and to use it in efficient ways. After people learn Qi Gong to the highest level, their bodies will have a stratum of luminosity, especially, the head will have a halo.

This can be seen by people, as long as they are calm and focused.

Coincidentally, Catholic artists paint Jesus, Mary, the angel, saints, and apostles with a halo on the head, and Buddhists paint or build Buddha's statue with a halo, too. No matter how they got this idea in the beginning, the same fact is that all these saints or Buddha have more powerful energy in their bodies, either through their own training or given by God.

Now we have learned the whole treatment procedure. This method can heal many diseases; the difference is in the timing, and needs determination to keep on practicing every day, then recovery can be expected.

After a person learns Qi Gong to a high level, if he does anal intercourse with someone of the same sex, he will feel repulsion between them, and then will understand the relationship between AIDS and anal intercourse.

CHAPTER 8

ADVICE FOR HOMOSEXUAL AND AIDS

PATIENTS

We have learned that AIDS is caused originally from anal intercourse, and the same way by physical and chemical means, we will infer that sexual relations between close relatives, such as parent and children or brother and sister, is considered an anti-natural law. Previously, except for moral or religious regulation, people could not prove this kind of sexual relationship was wrong scientifically; only from many cases the conclusion reached that marriage between close relatives could produce a deformed baby or retarded child. (Bad genes are reasons for deformities—Explained later in Questions & Answers – Question #46).

However, most regulations handed down from our ancestors usually belong to natural law. Until we can prove it is nonsense, we'd better just follow this as well. Especially, as living activities of our ancestors were very simple, most moral regulations came from experience which had accumulated for years, and conclusions were reached about what is right, what is wrong, what is allowed, and what is not allowed. This kind of accumulated experience is our cultural treasure; we should not give it up easily or foolishly, because this kind of behavior doesn't do us any good and just gives us more trouble such as AIDS. Furthermore, we can see such action as a kind of suicide.

Since human sexual behavior has existed since the beginning of humanity, it is very likely that ancient people knew as much as we do about sexual techniques. Therefore, we don't need to feel smart and infatuated with modern sexual art, especially in anal intercourse. People acquire more knowledge after reading a few ancient books, such as the Bible, Chinese medical books, the *Book of Changes* (I Qing), and the Buddhist Sutras. Other countries with long histories such as India, Iran and Egypt must have similar good books.

Since we are aware of the relationship between the human body and the magnetic field, by the inference process we may solve many disease problems that we previously couldn't. We may also understand the regulations handed down to us from ancient civilizations. Therefore, we do need to review the policy and purposes of all those regulations again, and to follow them more strictly, such as those against incest and against homosexual intercourse.

So we ask all people to cooperate, to quit these kinds of intercourse as soon as possible, for it is against natural law and will damage the human body, also to stop all kinds of activities that influence your people and others to do so, such as parades, demonstrations, advertisements and videotapes. Because young people are all curious and like to try anything new, especially if they've had drugs or alcohol, they may try them without any sense and so become addicted. Therefore, we should stop this kind of bad education to young people so that they don't even think about trying it. This would be my best reward for writing this book to help the people.

The author is also hoping that people will urge the government to set up a special research laboratory to do this kind of research, as mentioned before, to make it possible for more efficient and improved healing techniques and medicines to be developed soon. As for the patients unfortunately already affected by the AIDS virus, just don't be scared; currently they should be able to get healing from the way mentioned in the previous chapter.

If anyone has questions or needs the author's help, please write him a letter. He will try his best to answer. The email: **mingguocho15@gmail.com**.

CHAPTER 9

KEY POINTS IN THE PRACTICE OF QI GONG

Currently existing in the world, and handed down for generations, are many kinds of Qi Gong. Although they have different names, such as Qi Gong, Inner-Kong, Zen, Yoga, Meditation, Tai-Chi-Chuan, Sing-I-Chuan or Eight-Diagrams Chuan, actually they are all one base. It is: "By means of the magnetic field of the Sun, or moon, or earth or even living things, to induce or chafe the body's magnetic field to improve its volume of magnetic force" and then study how to apply it in martial art or medical healing or caring for health—further, to be a geomancer, astrologer or prophet. (quote—Explained later in this book – Question #47.)

So, while practicing Qi Gong, the best timing is before sunrise, because during that time: (1) the energy is refilled after sleeping, (2) the practice will let the extra energy be absorbed by the body, and (3) make every part of the body get stronger. That's why most books teaching Qi Gong recommend the practice not to be done during the daytime and midnight.

However, in the High Level Qi Gong, the book's teaching to practice right before 12 a.m. (noon) and after 12 p.m. (midnight) and mentions that are very important timing to get power or sphere (Dan)—those books' goals are to teach people to be the Holy Ghost with the human body, or so-called live Ghost. These kinds of people will not die and just be lifted to heaven like Jesus or Elijah (II Kings 2:11). This saying is very mysterious, but really can be found in books.

However, another reason to prohibit practicing at midnight is that, after practicing, people will be very vigorous and energetic, and find it hard to fall asleep.

Several books discuss methods of practice in more detail. They talk about different directions to face while practicing according to the seasons. Because this is very complicated, for the beginner, we may omit this temporarily. However, the many regulations again remind us of the close relationship between the human body and magnetic field; they prove once again that in the body there is magnetic induction.

Therefore, before beginning practice of Qi Gong, first of all, we should have a concept: the phenomenon is just like when people turn off the key of the car's motor but forget to turn off the lights: the battery's power will be used up very soon. But, before it is completely gone, if people want to start the motor again, they should turn off all other switches such as lights, air conditioner, radio, fan, and wait about five minutes for the battery to adjust itself and recover a little power. This concept is very important. Then, if the key is turned on, usually it will work. On the contrary, if this procedure is not followed, especially not turning off the air conditioner (which uses a lot of power at the same time), then there is no way that the car will start unless someone comes and recharges the battery.

So when people are starting to practiced Qi Gong, no matter which faction they belong to, the teacher always instructs: calm down, get rid of everything from the mind, think of nothing except concentrating on the sphere field, meaning turn off all unnecessary switches to conserve energy. Also, the sitting position must be very natural, body not bent nor twisted; be sure each part of each muscle is relaxed. The principle is to pile every piece of bone one upon another; even without muscle the structure won't collapse. That purpose is also to conserve energy. Maintaining this sitting or

70

standing position, after clearing out all unnecessary thoughts from the mind, then concentrate all attention on the sphere field (for the beginner, just concentrating on the position two inches below the navel will be fine). In the meantime, most of the energy in the whole body will go back to the sphere field (the body's battery).

This concept and method are easy to describe, yet difficult to do. Usually people will either fall asleep or lots of thoughts will keep coming up into their minds and they will lose themselves in thinking. So the Buddha always suggests that people murmur "Ah-Mi-Tol-Fo" (the name of Buddha) just as Catholic people murmur "In the name of the Father, the Son and the Holy Spirit." They say that God will help at the same time. Actually, I found that the only purpose is to help people to concentrate their minds. Therefore, if they repeat, "one, two, three, four" or "in, out" according to their breathing, it will help the same. Yet, don't do anything like "one through a thousand," because energy will be wasted or attention will get lost in thinking about the next figure to come up.

After acknowledging this concept, people will understand why, during the practice of Qi Gong, one has to obey such principles as follows:

(1)....Be sure all the muscles are relaxed: a slightly concave chest (not thrust forward), with straight back (neither bowed down nor the opposite); draw back the chin (don't face upward); drop the shoulders (many beginners will shrug instead). When sitting cross-legged, use any of several ways to cross the legs, as long as it is comfortable and can be maintained for a period of time, usually as pictured below:

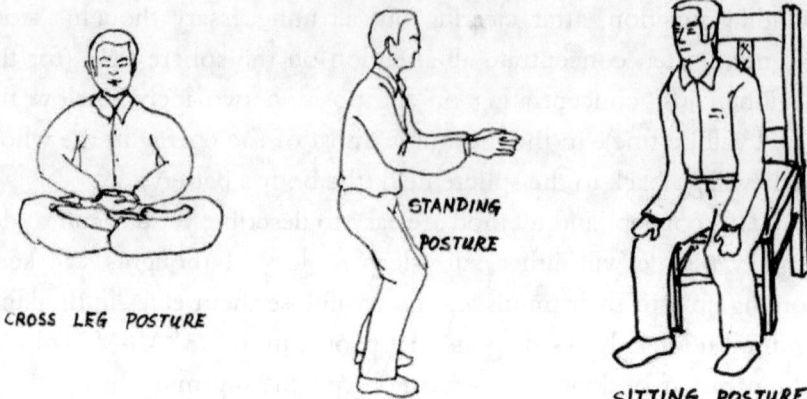

Figure 6

In the sitting posture, be sure the legs are straight down; both feet must be on the floor. The chair must be the same height as the lower leg's length or one to two inches higher so that the angle of the knees will be a little more than 90 degrees.

Qi Gong may also be done in a standing posture (shown above).

(2)…Relax the breathing: it must be natural and long and controlled, looking as if one is not inhaling.

(3)…Concentrate the mind solely on the sphere field.

(4)…Practice either before sunrise or after sunset.

(5)…It is better to practice with an empty stomach. One glass of warm water or warm milk is suggested. If the stomach is full, one may be wasting energy during digestion. Moreover, because one tries to draw energy to the sphere field, the energy supply to the stomach won't be enough, and can cause indigestion.

(6)…Don't eat icy cold food or drinks. Don't eat non-kosher food, especially pork, because most of these will increase resistance in the body.

(7)…Reduce times of sexual contact. Patients, during the first three months, must omit it entirely. Sexual excretions will be likely to draw out electrolytes from the battery and the power of the battery (sphere field) will become very weak.

(8)…Don't take a cold water bath. Practicing in an air conditioned room is prohibited absolutely. All the clothes must be loose and cover all the body, not only to prevent cold or rheumatism, but because while practicing, magnetism will go back into the sphere field, so that most parts of the body will be unprotected by magnetism, and become very weak. That also is the reason why, after one to two months practice, people will get colds easier than before.

(9)…In the beginning, each time, people need to practice at least 15 to 20 minutes, twice a day (early morning and night). When another new style is learned, then take an additional ten minutes. Later on, practice time may be extended as desired. Usually, after one month, people will need one hour to finish each time.

(10)…Practice every day, without skipping a day.

(11)…Learn with a good teacher.

All these are basic requirements. If one can practice without interruption for 30 days, one should have a sense about the existence of Qi and the Qi-sphere's movement; then, in the following days, one will improve very fast.

The experiment of sense about Qi: Everyone, no matter whether he has learned or not, will be able to sense it. If anyone wants to try, he may raise both hands up straight, about one minute, then drop the hand slowly; he may then sense the blood and Qi flowing down to the fingers. He will feel the hands and fingers slowly expand, a little numbed; sometimes, a few points on the hands (those are acupuncture points) will have a pulse beating. Those are a sense of Qi.

As a matter of fact, Chinese medical theory said, "Blood is carrying; Qi is guarding." It is emphasized that the force to move blood comes from the magnetism of the sphere, not from the heart. That's why acupuncture can staunch bleeding and do anesthesia. Scientists also wonder about the giraffe, whose neck is so long: how can a heart supply blood that high? The reason is the same.

So, even though the heart is still beating, yet many patients are in paralysis or monoplegia (paralysis of one muscle, extremity or muscle area). These kinds of symptoms occur because the magnetic force has been blocked or mislead, causing the blood to be unable to flow through to the place where it is needed, so that in that part of the body, tissue may become gangrenous. Another example is: when a man's penis cannot have an erection, the blood is circulating in it, but the magnetism is not enough. There are many reasons for this. After people learn Qi Gong for one year, the teacher may teach them how to control this too. "Yin Diau Gong" is the typical one of that function.

On the contrary, even if the heart is not beating, as long as the sphere field has enough power, the whole body still can get energy supplied from the sphere field so that the blood will not become congealed. This is the "Turtle-sleeping method," a kind of hi-level Qi Gong, similar to some animals' hibernation. This method can let people (not dead) go without eating or drinking for a few weeks or months. Today, the medical surgeon can change a person's heart successfully; the reasons are the same. Therefore, just as with a motor, turning the key off does not mean this car is junk; but, when the power of the battery is used up, the car will not start unless the battery is recharged. When the battery is totally dead, then the motor must get a new battery.

CHAPTER 10

CONCLUSION

We have used most chapters to discuss AIDS because the author found that the public's perceptions about AIDS and homosexual behavior already have gone into the wrong direction in research. Unless we review and change it right away, billions of dollars in treatment and research will be wasted, plus timing and manpower. Moreover, many more AIDS patients will not get cures in time. Therefore, we cannot but emphasize it in this book.

何大一：每天有6300人染愛滋

記者黃子怡／劍橋市報導

波士頓台灣人生物科技學會（BTBA）14日在哈佛大學科學院館舉辦研討會。著名愛滋專家何大一等三位專家發表專題演講，有300餘名年輕學生學者參與盛會，會中並提供求職講座與機會。

愛滋專家何大一院士目前主導洛克菲勒大學（Rockefeller University）所屬的艾倫戴蒙愛滋研究中心（The Aaron Diamond AIDS Research Center）。何大一介紹愛滋病現狀，並給予投身研究的年輕學者建議。

何大一說，全球有3500萬人死於愛滋病，另外同等人數罹患愛滋病，每天有6300人感染，即使有充分的資金與人力，30年來的研究仍然無法生產疫苗，因為愛滋病毒的結構讓抗生素無法發揮效用。

但是，何大一指出，目前仍在研究階段的抗生素Ibalizumab與人體免疫系統中的CD4受體結合，可防止愛滋病毒侵入細胞。何大一表示，雖然愛滋病最初在同性戀族群發現，但感染率高的非洲大多數為異性戀者。在中國，愛滋病例集中於都會，如瀋陽和北京。何大一說，防止愛滋感染的教育是必要措施，

但醫學界不會批判病人行為。

對與剛起步的學者們，何大一給予寶貴建議。他鼓勵大家往自己所熱愛的方向前進，在思考和行動中找到平衡。勇於接受挑戰，發展必要的知識與技術，在尋找真相的過程中，能夠挑戰虛偽的權威。

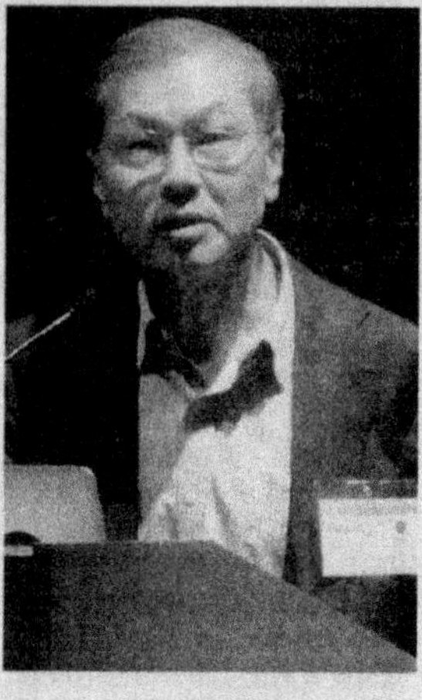

何大一說明全球有7000萬人受愛滋病影響。 （記者黃子怡／攝影）

Figure 7

The article was from a speech at BTBA in Harvard University Science Building on 6-14-2014.

The previous paragraph was written 25 years ago. And today, Dr. Ho of Aaron Diamond AIDS Research Center of Rockefeller University said, "There are thirty five million people who have died of AIDS. Besides, there is still the same amount of people sick with AIDS who are waiting for treatment. An average of 6300 people is contracting AIDS every day. Although there is enough financial and manpower support after 30 years of research, we still cannot produce an efficient vaccine because the structure of the AIDS virus disable the functions of the antibiotics." Is that statement enough to prove what the author said: "the perceptions about AIDS already have gone in the wrong direction in research." And finally, Dr. Ho suggested, "People should develop the necessary knowledge and technique to look for the truth, so that can challenge the existent authority." This is the purpose of this book. Would they accept my proposals humbly?

However, after the reader finishes this book, he will find the major purpose of this book is to emphasize this new idea to the public and to the medical industry:

1)…The human body is an electromagnetic body and magnetism is in and out of the whole body.

2)…There is a battery, the sphere field, in the human body.

The author realizes that his analyses and explanations may not be one hundred percent clear. It would be difficult to understand them entirely, since so far, this concept about electric and magnetic energies is still based on all kinds of assumptions.

However, a very important fact is that in Oriental clinical experience the Qi Gong has been developed to a perfect system. Although the special phrases the Chinese used are totally incompatible with modern science, yet we need to understand that the Qi Gong system was founded and developed thousands of years ago. During that time, people did not have any idea about electric and magnetic, so they developed a usable system or theory totally based on practical experience. Therefore, if we follow the track which ancient people developed, definitely we will find the same result. Moreover, we will be very much surprised to find that most of the ancient Chinese knowledge all came from Qi Gong. (All knowledge?—Explained later in this book – Question #48.) Qi Gong developed the *Book of Changes* (the I Qing 3000 years ago), Chinese Zen (using three fingers in taking the pulse to diagnose where and what illness is in the body). Even the Heaven and Hell concepts, which developed in India and China (ancient Egypt), were based on

Qi Gong principles and experience (Question #49).

The author found that the reason Qi Gong did not take root in western countries is that western culture mostly comes from the Bible, and the Bible has many prohibitions about getting involved with those mysteries. A major point is that God does not want people to get involved with those mysteries because, if we are to trust Him, we may leave everything to Him and don't need to be too smart or to worry about the future (some will question this theory— Explained later in this book.). A typical example in the Bible is that God didn't want the Jewish people to have their own king because God is their king, so when the Jewish people asked for a king, God was not happy; that was a kind of insult to God. (How wanting a king relates to Qi Gong—Explained later in this book – Question #50).

However, it is a fact that, since all the mysteries are based on Qi Gong, if we can develop it as a science, then today's science will have achieved completion.

This is also the reason, not only for AIDS patients, that many cancers, stroke or paralysis patients who are deemed impossible to cure, turn to an Oriental-trained doctor, and usually get cured or at least much improved. If somebody did not recover, the fault is not in the system but in the practioner. So far, no one organization has emerged with the knowledge, resources, and power to handle and systematically reorganize Oriental medical science, and to re-evaluate the entire medical personally, and then divide them into groups. Therefore, many beginners can pretend to be great doctors without basis. Consequentially, sometimes there are cases of mistreatment in Oriental medicine as well as there are cases of malpractice in western medicine. The author, therefore, sincerely asks that science and the public re-examine their theories and be willing to include the valuable treasure of Oriental culture in their thinking. Not to do so would be a tragedy in human history.

The previous paragraph was written by 1989. As a matter of fact, after a few years practice up to 2014, the author had found:

1...Mesothelioma is not a cancer. It had nothing to do with

asbestos, can be relieved overnight, and can be cured within weeks. The author was asbestos certified by New York State (Certificate # 10-10166 and New York City Department of Environmental Protection CRS 1195530-Expires 10/9/2012).

2…Most cancers (tumors) can be cured within a short time (3 to 12 months) and at a low cost ($2,000 to $24,000). The causes and treatment can be gotten from page 21 to page 175 of surgery in textbook *Yi-Chong-Gin-Gieng* (medical textbook: Golden Rules). It was published 500 years ago.

3…Lupus is not one disease, but is hundreds of diseases, depending on where (meridians, skin, muscle, bones, and organs) and what (air bubble—Chinese called it wind, ANA showed up; heat or fever—ds DNA showed up; moisture or water—medical report says rheumatic, yet no specific lab test figure can be seen.) in there, and most can be cured within 3 months. My patient in Missouri who was cured by the author is proof with medical report evidence and a doctor as a witness. All these proofs can be seen from the Attorney General's office file. (That means the author did not lie based on the government's proof.)

4…Most of the pain killers caused the lawsuit for a billion dollars because their side effects were wrong. Without those pain killers, the symptoms will happen eventually. Doctors don't know that. Pharmacists and the pharmaceutical companies don't know that; lawyers don't know that; and judges don't know that. What a catastrophe. What a chaos. Not only poor people cannot afford, but also rich people waste their money and suffer until they finally die. So, government will go bankrupt eventually.

5…Alzheimer's and M.S. (multiple sclerosis) are caused from acupuncture points were hit during certain timing, so the "Qi" (life energy) was blocked to being delivered to the brain (Alzheimer's) or muscle (M.S.) See previous pages how the Heart Meridian controls the brain 11 a.m.-3 p.m., and Spleen Meridian controls muscles during 9 a.m.-11 a.m.

6…The misjudgment of oriental herbs. Such as:

a…Rhinoceros horn is good for lupus, but has nothing to do with sex. The horn was prohibited from being sold in order to protect the species, but what about using a dead rhinoceros's horn?

b…Prepared aconite root is the only herb to cure leukemia as long as one removes the skin and peduncle. Then the poison will be gone and safe to be taken. It was prohibited from being sold in the market by the FDA.

c…Immature bitter orange is very good for mesothelioma, but do not use more than three pieces at a time. It is not for long-term intake. It was prohibited from being sold in the markets by the FDA, and the doctor said this disease is not curable.

d…Ephedra herb is very good for the first stage of lupus (numbness and stiffness of neck and shoulders). Doctors said this disease had to do with the bones (thorn).

e…Ginkgo nut has nothing to do with memory. It is good for coughing, bladder control, kills bacteria, and may "reduce phlegm." This function will make people's mind clearer, so western company doctors claim it can improve memory. An overdose can make women's menstrual period irregular. Also, eating around 100 pieces will kill people overnight. So, the FDA said that herb is not good and blamed the herbal treatment.

CHAPTER 11

A FEW CASES OF NON-MEDICAL HEALING

UNDER THE GUIDANCE OF THE AUTHOR

(1988)

After readers finish the previous ten chapters, the author believes that most readers will be wondering, "Who is this author and how dare he touch this big problem of healing?" What the author can say is that even he, himself, is surprised that his talent is on mechanical functions. Fortunately, by coincidence the author got a chance to learn a little bit about those kinds of knowledge that most people think is nonsense, so he was urged by curiosity to find out whether they are false or true. Because he is the kind of person who neither trusts nor abandons anything very easily unless he has good proof, this even includes his religion, although his grandfather and uncles are pastors. So this enabled him to find that among all the different mysteries there is something related; all are somewhat unexpectedly based on the principles that are mostly in Qi Gong.

The author has been able to apply his knowledge of these basic principles to affect a number of physical cures. Several brief case histories follow.

Case 1: The author's wife, Grace, age 39, born in 1951.

When she married the author, she was 25 years old. At that time, she was very weak and there was a yellow mottle in the white of her eye. Every day when she came home from her office, she was tired, sleepy, had a poor appetite, and felt nauseous. A doctor's examination showed that her liver was weak, similar to hepatitis. The doctor said that the only way to recover was resting often and eating more nutritious food. She followed his instructions for three years, but nothing improved.

The author had insisted that she should not take any medicine to avoid pregnancy. When she was 28, finances were better and we were ready to have a baby. Yet, for one year, nothing happened. So we both decided to go to Brooklyn Hospital to check for any problems. After checking, the doctor said the author was all right, and then concentrated on checking Grace. For almost six months, she took all kinds of tests and treatments, still nothing. Finally, the doctor suggested a small operation, but the author refused because nothing was guaranteed. Then the case was dropped for a while. Meanwhile, Grace and the author were praying very sincerely for a miracle.

One day, Mr. Wang, the husband of Grace's sister, introduced us to a Chinese female doctor, Dr. Hwa-Qing Wu. She was an associate professor at the Chinese medical and herbal college in Taiwan. She had written a book called *Chinese Medical Science of the Female*.

Dr. Wu came to New York to apply for her daughter's immigration from mainland China. She stayed temporarily in Chinatown waiting for information. Meanwhile, she also rented a small herbal store to diagnose and treat patients (1980).

She used the three-finger method to take Grace's pulse in both wrists for about ten minutes, an oriental system which provides a check of the vital organs as well as the heartbeat. Dr. Wu said that both Grace's liver and spleen were not functioning right, and also showed in the eye white with the yellow mottle, the organic weakness leaves the uterus with little power to hold the fertilized ovum; the ovum, even if fertilized, would flow out and Grace couldn't get pregnant. However, if the liver and spleen were healed, and they recovered their functions, she could become pregnant easily.

The author asked the doctor how long it would take to get pregnant; she said about three to four months. So Grace started to take the treatments with Dr. Wu. Her way was to give acupuncture once a week for about one hour each time. After the acupuncture, we took a 7-day supply of herbs and went home to make herb tea to drink twice a day. The fee was $10 a day.

After four months, Grace's health was a little better; the color of the mottle in her eye white became lighter, yet there was no sign of pregnancy. Usually people would just give up or even sue the doctor for fraud. However, we thought, if Grace's health could recover, why not give the treatment more time? Although the author did not keep all the records about the prescriptions, he knows the doctor did change the medicine many times according to what Grace's response was. Finally, ten months later, the yellow mottle was very light and Grace's appetite was much better. The doctor said it was time for the pregnancy. In the eleventh month after starting this doctor's treatment, Grace became pregnant. The next year we had a baby girl and gave her the Chinese name, Nai-En, which means "it is grace."

Although Grace's health had recovered enough to have a baby, yet it was much worse than that of the average person. For instance, when she was discharged from the hospital three days after the delivery, she could not get off the bed by herself and had to have someone hold her.

In another year and a half, we had another baby girl and gave her the Chinese name, Siau-En, which means "Appreciate Grace." We joked, saying, "Buy one, get one free," referring to the idea of getting a second baby from the treatments.

After the second daughter was born, because it was two times after delivery, the author started to pay a lot of attention to caring for Grace when she was confined. She became very strong, ate more, and could work longer than the author did. Then it was the author's turn to be cared for by her.

Five years later, the author got a secret formula from a friend—"HOW TO HAVE A BABY BOY OR GIRL." IT SAID: WHEN MAKING LOVE, IF THE MALE EJECTS SPERM WHEN THE FEMALE REACHES HER CLIMAX OR AFTER, THE BABY WILL BE A BOY. IF THE FEMALE DOES NOT REACH HER CLIMAX, THE BABY WILL BE A GIRL.

After reviewing ourselves, the author found it was right: before the first pregnancy, Grace was so weak she had no sexual appetite; before the second pregnancy, because the first baby had just stopped breast feeding, Grace was very busy with the baby and her health had not recovered, so she was listless.

Therefore, after a discussion, we were willing to try one more time, following the formula. We were very careful to make sure Grace was in climax every time, especially in those days from the fourth day after the end of the menses for the next two weeks.

Exactly as we expected, the next year we had a baby boy. His Chinese name, Zon En, means "Glory to the grace." At that time, Grace was 38 years old and very healthy. In the hospital, the first day after delivery, she already could get off the bed by herself. From this case, the author can reach a few conclusions.

a)…From his successful experience with the formula of female climax, the author believes that with orgasm, there is a special secretion from somewhere, maybe the oviduct, womb or vagina, and that this is acting against the sperm, carrying the female chromosome. Otherwise, the regular secretion in the female's sexual organs may be acid so that the male chromosome carrying the sperm will be stopped or killed and the female sperm will survive.

This would be the same as the way often used to have a baby boy: using a 0.2% soda solution to wash the vagina before making love, recorded as about 70%-80% successful. If scientists can get this special secretion from women, before and after orgasm, then this assumption can be proved.

b)…If the previous assumption can be proved, then it will show the male and female essential qualities' differences since the sperm will be alkaline suitable or acid suitable. So, the man or woman getting married is a case of neutralization by acid and alkali in chemistry.

c)…From (b), we can get further evidence that homosexual intercourse is against natural law.

One more example happened with Grace. About a month after the baby boy was born, one night in the middle of March the temperature dropped to single digits Fahrenheit in New York City, and it just happened that night that the furnace was not working in the house. The portable heater was not enough, and the temperature in the house dropped to about 20 degrees or less. The next day, Grace developed a headache. The author realized that a cold air had blown into her head one month after delivery. Without a very good treatment, this could be a lifetime ailment. A western doctor would tell her to take aspirin, but that would cope with only the symptoms, and would not get rid of the source of the ailment. So the author took her to Chinatown to the owner of a Chinese herbal store, who was also an herbal doctor. We took about two weeks doses of herbal medicine home to make herbal tea. In about three weeks, the headache was gone completely. This was another example that somehow the cold gets into the Qi-vascular and make more resistance for the Qi to pass through, so that causes the headache. We knew to be cautious about her headache, because Grace's mother has suffered with a side headache all her life since her last delivery thirty years ago.

Case 2: A Female Patient

The author had a Chinese restaurant in midtown Manhattan near Fifth Avenue called Grace Restaurant. Most customers are well-to-do. One lady, a frequent customer for about two years, had started using two canes instead of one to walk and seemed to be getting worse.

One day, the author asked her if there might be a way he could help. She said she needed a good doctor and a good lawyer in order to reinstate the medical insurance that had just been canceled.

She had been hit by a truck while riding a bicycle several years before and the cartilage between the femur and pelvis had been damaged and was wearing away. Walking was very painful. Four times every day, she had to take large doses of pain killers and four times a week she went to physical therapy, just to be able to continue to work.

The author told her his help did not mean getting a lawyer because even if the case would be won, the painkillers could not help her recover. Also, taking painkillers too long will damage the body, hurting the kidneys, liver or causing addiction.

Therefore, the author found a Chinese acupressure (massage) doctor in Queens. Every day at 4 p.m., the author took her to this doctor for acupressure therapy, and brought her back home, altogether about three hours a day. The extra effort was appropriate for several reasons: the customer had become a good friend, the doctor did not speak English, the treatment was expensive and the taxi would also be very expensive, since she could not use the subway or bus. The author also wanted to evaluate how good the doctor was and to be sure that the patient would not give up too soon, before the therapy had a chance to work.

The first day after the therapy, this lady could stand without canes for a few minutes. One week after following the doctor's instructions, she could stop taking painkillers. Every day for about a month, she felt better and better, and could walk a few more steps without her canes.

Meanwhile, because the restaurant was getting into its busy season, the author could not continue going with her, so he suggested that she find an acupressure doctor in midtown. He also suggested some special physical therapy exercises she could do at home. The following letter accompanied a dictionary (*New Medical Lexicon*):

"To Mr. Mingguo Cho

A tiny token of deepest thanks and appreciation for the extraordinary kindness that lifted me out of despair and put me into recovery.

No American doctor would do so much. Some have made partial attempts, but none really believed it possible.

You have proved I could be well, and it is happening.

All praise and thanks to you.

The enclosed is a start of your medical library for your future medical treatment center that combines Eastern and Western medical systems.

The time is right for this; I think you should do it.

Then you can heal many people who might not otherwise be healed, and make many people very happy.

You have a gift for healing that not even many doctors have, and it deserves to be realized. Let's begin now to let your excellent idea become a reality."

Sincerely,

Mary Ann Carroll

The reason the author dared to attempt this test for recovery was from the idea of Qi Gong. He though that even though her cartilage was damaged and mixed with hematoma, if she could get the right therapy, one way to pull the bones off each other a little bit, the other way, the Qi will go inside the space between the two bones. That will take the cartilage's place and help a little like an air cushion.

This is the same reason the baby's bone joints can bend much more than the adult's can. Senior people will be worse because their Qi is less than young people's, so the space between bones becomes closer and closer. If they go to learn Qi Gong, it will help them get back toward the baby's style. For examples of that, you may see many senior people in the park where Chinese practice Tai-Gi-Chuan.

Case 3: The author's grandfather, age 90 (1998)

A rugby player in high school and very healthy, the author's grandfather was a pastor for most of his life. Now he is in a nursing home in Texas, with hands and feet very stiff, almost paralytic, and having lost most of his memory. The author, after discussion with his uncle, asked his uncle to send the grandfather from Texas to the author's house in New York. An acupuncturist came every morning to give treatment and the author gave a bed bath and foot acupressure treatment at night. Meanwhile, the author also gave him a kind of Chinese medicine every day to improve the Qi channel's flow, but he could only take a little, as it was mostly vomited out. In addition, the author's mother and aunt fed and entertained the grandfather, sometimes singing or telling stories, trying to bring back his thoughts.

After one week, there was obvious improvement; the grandfather was willing to talk, he played Go, a Chinese chess game, with the author, and could remember to put the stones on the board, but couldn't concentrate to analyze the paths of thought. On the ninth day, he cried loudly all of a sudden, and seemed to have a kind of melancholia with mixed self-obstruction and frustrated. Because he was the oldest in the family and never would talk about his problems with anyone because of pride; therefore he became out of his mind. So all the methods to help were to relax him and bring him back to reality. However, the doctor said it would be very difficult, because after a period of treatment, he would become depressed and revert to negative thoughts. Because the patient would repeat the same cycle of thinking again and again, especially at his age, it was very difficult to stimulate him and keep him interested.

We worked until the twelfth day and could see a steady improvement, but then he caught a cold with a fever of 104 degrees.

The author had to send him to the hospital, because no one else in the family was professional enough to take care of him, and the author's business hours in the restaurant ranged from 11 a.m. to 10:30 p.m.

While he was in the hospital for one week, the author and the acupuncture doctor were not allowed to treat him, so by the time of discharge, his condition just went back to what it formerly was, except for the "cold." Then, because the restaurant business went into another season, the author could not do it anymore, so the grandfather went back to the nursing home in Texas.

Although this was not a successful case, the author still could see the improvement made by his idea.

That was in 1998, later on, similar symptoms happened on his tenant. She fell on the staircase and hurt her wrist. The wrist was swollen. Then within two weeks, she started to forget where her keys, money, and passport were. It turned out to be "Alzheimer's." And this reminded the author that his grandfather had fallen on the street and forgot how to go home. The people who brought him home found him on the ground and wanted to remove the rock which tripped him. And later on, he was just standing besides the wall murmuring.

These two cases let the author find out that "Alzheimer's" somehow related to the fall on the wrist, which the author had discussed in another paper, similar to how M.S. (Multiple Sclerosis) was found. Both of them belong to the illness due to being hit at the acupuncture points. (2013)

The causes and treatment to cure are also found in the Chinese book of Martial Arts: Alzheimer is caused by hitting on the point of Sen Men (Spirit Gate) point (belongs to the heart meridian) and the heart meridian connects to the brain and controls the memory. The M.S. is caused by hitting on the Zhang Men point (belongs to the liver meridian) or the point of Fu-Ai (belongs to the spleen meridian); the liver controls the tendons, the spleen controls the muscles. And still, the hitting time is another key point, for Alzheimer, most of the time was hit during lunch time (11 a.m. to 1 p.m.). For the liver meridian (Zhang Men) was hit during midnight (1 a.m. to 3 a.m.); for the spleen meridian (Fu-Ai) was hit during the morning (9 a.m. to 11 a.m.). If these illnesses were not solved in the proper way, it would take a long time to shrink, then paralysis. Can our American insurance system afford to cover such costs? Note: If the hitting time is not during the time period, the illness will not be that serious.

Case 4: The author's mother-in-law, age 65

About six years previously, her son had immigrated to New York, having just learned Qi Gong from Master Wu San-Chu. He had learned very well and knew it was very good for health, so he started to teach his mother. She was a good student, too, and for six years she practiced faithfully. For more than thirty years, she had suffered severe headaches which had started when she had a cold after her last childbirth, and she could never recover, just like what the author's wife, Grace, had. However, after these years practicing Qi Gong, she seems much better.

Last year, she went for a complete checkup. The doctor is a very good western doctor and is also our church's Presbyter. After all kinds of tests, the doctor found symptoms of liver cancer, and all the reports pointed to that. However, after a microscopic examination of the affected tissues that were cut into very thin pieces, the doctor determined there was no more cancer. All the documents are still in the doctor's file.

We all attributed the recovery to her son, because he taught her Qi Gong six years before. That way, even the cancer cells stopped developing and she started on the way to recovery.

In her case, the author had wondered a long time already whether she had a liver problem too, because her face color was dark, like over-burnt. Also, she had continuously taken too much medication over thirty years for the headaches, which would definitely hurt her liver. Yet, the author couldn't say anything, because he was not sure. He, himself, was learning Qi Gong almost at the same time as she was.

From the previous four cases, although there is nothing related to AIDS, they are nevertheless based on the Chinese medical theory, and if we delve deeply into them, whether acupuncture, acupressure, pulse study Zen, even the herbal book, we will find they are all based on Qi Gong. So, from Qi Gong to review the body, then the author had the idea about the body's magnetic field and the body's battery, the "sphere field," and from that he deduced that the etiology of AIDS must have something to do with the destruction of the magnetic field and the sphere field.

Though the author is not a specialist in any industry, fortunately he is a semi-specialist in many industries, including architecture, auto mechanics, Qi Gong, Religion, Chinese and western medicine, so that he is able to write this book and combine these specialties. Yet, because he is just a semi-specialist, (he already proved himself by 2015 superior to some medical specialists), all he can do is use this book to tell the public that he has already found a gold mine in the medical industry. With regard to how we can mine that gold, it will depend on all kinds of specialists sharing their knowledge.

The previous draft was done by 1988. Since there was no official medical document as proof, the author's idea could not be deemed serious. And the author saw many relatives die: his sister-in-law died of breast cancer; the other sister-in-law died of uterine cancer; and his mother-in-law died from liver problems.) Two famous Chinese singers died of AIDS (before they died, the author predicted they were going to die from AIDS, because both of them were active gay men.) It turned out: one committed suicide by jumping from a tall building, though some rumored he murmured: "why did it happened to me?" after he saw the medical report. However, his lover was still alive and active. We know he is a good singer, actor, and a good man, loyal to his lover—so the medical report never officially mentioned what disease he had for privacy reasons. The other one was sent to the hospital for the reason (in newspapers) of liver cancer and died there. But from the photo, the author could see he did not have liver cancer, because his skin was always white, not dark brown that happens with liver cancer patients. Also, his face shrank very much and lost his charming looks. People may challenge the author by saying that was too arbitrary without evidence. However, "to see something is to say something." All the truth was hidden in the name of privacy. How can a doctor do the research? That forced the author to go another way.

CHAPTER 12

A FEW CASES OF NON-MEDICAL AND MEDICAL HEALING UNDER THE TREATMENT OF THE AUTHOR (INCLUDES AIDS PATIENT, LUPUS PATIENT, MESOTHELIOMA PATIENT AND HIGH CHOLESTEROL PATIENT UP TO 2013)

(I)… Qi Gong self-healing
(a)…For burnt skin

The author is an architectural engineer, so most of the time he repaired his own car and his house. One time he repaired his flat roof because it was leaking. He did not wear gloves. After making the repairs, his hands had been stained with a little tar. He went to the kitchen to clean his hands. As people know, tar is not easy to remove. He decided to try carburetor cleaner. When he sprayed it on his hands, right away the tar dissolved and was gone little by little. So, he gladly kept on spraying. All of a sudden, fire shot from the pilot light under the stove top to his hands. His two hands became torches. The kitchen cabinets also caught fire. He was shocked, but managed to put his hands under the faucet to flush the chemical off. Because a little tar was still attached to his hand, that still burned under the running water. Finally, the fire was extinguished after he put his hands in a bucket of water.

After that, he had to go out to spray his hands until the tar was gone. But very soon, the skin of his hands swelled with water bubbles. The author had to use a needle to pierce and let out the secretion, so the skin could protect the muscle. However, two spots with thick tar kept on burning until he had put his hands in water had no bubbles, but became like charcoal.

He treated his hands with Vaseline a few times every day. After about five days, most of his hands were back to normal. However, the two charcoal spots remained the same—no feeling and a dark brown color. Some friends said he may need a skin graft from skin taken at the hip.

Because the author was busy and had no medical insurance, he did not go to the hospital. Instead, he practiced Tai-Chi Qan a few times every day. After one week, he started to have feelings at the injured spots: feelings were like hundreds of needles pierced the edge of the charcoal skin. It did not hurt. There was itching, but comfortable. I knew the "Qi" was having its healing effects. So, I practiced Tai-Chi more and even concentrated on the two hands too. Qi Gong healing may be conducted by the healer to focus on the injured parts (location), so the Qi (energy) will go there in order to affect healing. Then, feeling remained the same, but the dark brown spots were getting smaller and smaller. About three months later, the two spots disappeared and the skin became normal. The two black skin spots never peeled off. Instead, they just changed their color and look like new skin came where the dead skin had been.

(b)…For broken tendon

Years ago, one Sunday after church: one of our church members had a small car that was blocked by two other cars after she parked on the street side. There was no way to drive it out. After half an hour of waiting, we decided to remove the car sideways by lifting it with our hands. The author and three others members held the four ends of the front and back bumpers, then lifted the car up and down inch by inch to move it from right to left. We called out, "One, two three." to keep coordinated in our efforts. But the last one the author seems did it himself and did not know why the other three put the car down at the same time with most of the weight on the author's hand. He felt a small pop sound in his finger. He knew something was wrong—his middle finger's tendon was injured—injured, but not completely broken.

Later on, his middle finger was starting to swell the size of a hot dog. He did not have medical insurance and could not afford to go to the hospital, Every morning his finger looked like a hot dog. What he could do was to rub his finger only, from the upper section to the palm. Then until the evening, the finger reduced its swelling. Besides the rubbing therapy, the author also bought an herbal tea from a Chinese store to help the rubbing. It took about half a year to recover completely.

(c)…An example of one AIDS patient with Qi Gong training.
Witness: brother of the patient, Cerorclo Esteban (718-937-8520).
Patient's name: Jorge Esteban. D.O.B.: 4/23/1963
He has since died. Former address: 83-05 34th Avenue, Jackson Heights, NY 11370
Hospitals: St. Vincent's Hospital   Doctor: James Mazzara
               Elmhurst Hospital   Doctor: Alonso

Around 12/27/94. Through Mr. Edgardo Cardinari's (Editor of *Noticias del Mundo*) arrangement, the author had a chance to have the audience of around 100. Then about 20 AIDS patients were willing to join the free Qigong Training Class. After three months of training, only one patient graduated. Others gave up, either they were too bored to practice alone or too busy to take time to practice. Mr. Jorge Esteban was the one who graduated. He had AIDS since 1990. He started the seminar on 12/27/1994 and was brought there by his brother. When he came to the seminar, his condition was that he could barely walk to the supermarket from home. His T4 count was 10, temperature was 109 F degrees already for 15 days. His sexual habit was heterosexual.

After 4 weeks of Qi Gong practice, His T4 cell count went from 10 and increased to 56 until 3/20/1995. His temperature was normal. He also had taken the doctors' medicine continuously.

Report: Total T cell   CD3 52%   (normal 70 ~ 80)

Helper T cell CD 4 2L%   (normal 30 ~ 56)

Supt   CD 8 49H%   (normal 15 ~ 35)

CD4/CD8   0.04L   (normal 1.5 ~ 1.7)

Absolute   CD 3   480

Absolute   CD 4   56   (normal 1000)

Absolute   CD8   450

He started to go back to English class (ESL) by himself. (Before that, he could not walk too far.)

He also started to practice boxing with his brother.

But one thing was no good: he had a new girlfriend from English class. That was a bad influence to his healthy recovery, because he could no longer keep growing his sperm level (due to his sexual lifestyle). Then until June, 1995, he had to go back to the hospital because of an emergency situation.

The first time when he went back to the hospital (6/17/1995), he felt scared, so he practiced Qi Gong very hard in the hospital. Then he recovered his energy very soon. He was discharged very soon. Again, for the second time he returned to the hospital on September, 1995 because he had recovered too fast. Even his doctor said to him, "I don't know what you did, but it seems it was very helpful to your recovery." Unfortunately, he depended on "Qi Gong" to absorb energy, but neglected to keep his "sperm" level. This wrong behavior killed him. When there is no more electrolyte fluid in the battery, no matter how long it has been charged (practice Qi Gong), the battery will be dead anyhow. So, he died In February, 1996.

This sad story ended the author's experiment. It sounds as if he had "failed." But readers can easily see the difference between before and after Qi Gong practice. And readers should be able to predict that, if Mr. Esteban did not have a new girlfriend so he could maintain and increase his sperm level and kept with his Qi Gong practice, he would be better and alive. The author has said: one hundred days of practice to build a Qi Gong foundation he had done. It would take three years of practice to reach the completion. By that amount of time, his sperm would be back to normal (both quality and volume). Then, the AIDS virus should have disappeared automatically and completely. We could then say the AIDS was cured. Be attention is "the volume level of sperm" is meant natural level without "sexual activity". Or said another way, "once every other month" because usually men will have "nocturnal pollution" once a month anyway. But beware again: If physical exercise is hard, the "nocturnal ejaculation" will be skipped and the sperm will be changed to "Qi" and "Qi" will be changed to bone material that make the density of bone stronger. Also, the bone marrow would be purified and produce good blood. That is what we really want and no ejaculation is the goal. These series of functions reverse when people are taking drugs. That is why with people who are taking drugs they seem to have a lot of energy especially in sexual activities or exercise. But later on, they become skinny and their bones become very fragile.

II...An Herbal Treatment:
(A)...Cure for LUPUS

LUPUS is considered incurable by all the doctors and considered the most complicated disease ever: Because LUPUS, just like a heat wave on earth, wherever it goes, will cause a fever—that will be shown on the ds DNA index. That can happen from head to toes, hands, and legs, outside in from the skin, muscle, tendon, bone, and inner organs.

The medical industry's treatment (medicine) include: (1) Prednisone which tries to separate antibodies from antigens so they won't fight each other to cause fever. That is very efficient, so most of the time the fever is reduced right away. But what causes the production of antigens has never been found. Then, the antigens kept on producing, so as the antibodies. It turned out were out of control by Prednisone, then the patients would die.

The other two medicines were (2) Mycophenolate mofeti and (3) Cyclosoprine.

The other medicine: (4) Chloroquine Phosphat is the treatment for the problem of feeling hot and cold repeatedly, just like the symptoms of malaria.

Other medicines were used just for treating the partial problem to relieve temporarily.

The author had a few successful cases, but that will be in another book—LUPUS, because this book is not focused on LUPUS. The author, although he has no medical background, he could achieve what the medical industry could not. So, he points out one typical case of LUPUS he cured within three months who was given up by the hospital, but he was sued by the patient with Consumer Affairs by the Missouri Attorney General. All the legal evidence is in the Attorney General's file, so the reader can check out the case to see that the author has not lied. (More details are in Foreword.)

From this case, the reader can see that the author did the following:

1...Never saw the patient, but treated her remotely—only depended on her medical report and her mother's oral description.

2...Reduced her high fever that was already out of control from taking Prednisone, but the fever reduced overnight just taking an herbal compound.

3...The patient had been under the doctor's treatment for 6 years and, only off and on, until out of control.

4...Cured her within three months.

The most interesting thing found: the case in the Bible of Job who was tested by Satan. Satan challenged God about Job's loyalty and so Job came down with a terrible disease—that is LUPUS. The author is proud to claim that he solved this mysterious disease completely. And he dares to accept any public challenge.

(B) Herbs to Treat "Mesothelioma"

"Mesothelioma" is considered a kind of horrible "cancer," and deemed related to "asbestos." Actually, the author found that "mesothelioma" is NOT A CANCER, because doctors could not find cancer cells at all.

And mesothelioma is NOT RELATED to asbestos. Its symptoms are the chest blows up, so the patient cannot breathe, has no appetite, but feels full and has pain in the chest. The <u>REAL CAUSES</u> is the fact that patient has LUPUS. In the procedure of treatments for regular lupus, it is recommended to let the patient sweat first, then vomit, and then have diarrhea. If in reverse or having a second process too early before the first process is completed, then the bad air would sometime mix with moisture and stay in the chest, could not come out, and that causes the problem. To treat this problem can be done overnight, but to cure the patient's LUPUS problem is another story.

The formulas of the herb's compound to treat are:

(A) Gathering in the chest: full feeling in the chest and pain, try to let the patient..diarrhea too early before sweating is the cause, having pain feeling, pulse is not obvious unless you press hard.

(a) Big gathering: from heart to belly, full fill with air, painful and not even touchable.

<u>Formula of herbs:</u> Rheum officinate baill (240 grams); Natrii Sulfas (60 grams); Lepidium Apetalum Willd (40 grams); Almond (40 grams); Kansui (4 grams).

<u>Cooking Method:</u> bring one quart of water to boil: add Officinale, Apetalum, Almond for 50 minutes (low fire) until 1/3 of herb tea is left; then remove those herbs from the pot; and put in Nutriio Sulfas for 3 minutes until they are dissolved. After removing the dirt, there are about 2 cups of herb tea left. Drink this tea; one cup with 2 grams of Kansui powder. Drink twice within 24 hours.

(b) Small gathering: a little air forms below the heart, not hungry, feels pain only under pressure.

<u>Formula of herbs:</u> Coptis Root (40 grams); Pinellia Tuber (40 grams); Trichosanthes (one piece sliced).

<u>Cooking Method:</u> boil the Trichosanthes in one quart of water on a low fire until half the volume (one pint) is left. Discard the sediment, then add the Coptis and Pinellia and cook for 15 minutes on a low fire. Discard the sediment again. There is 2/3 pint of tea left. Separate that for three portions. Drink every 8 hours.

(c) Air gathering with water: a little fever, sweating on the head, and full in the chest.

<u>Formula of herbs:</u> The same as (a) above, but add one soup spoon of honey while taking each time.

<u>Cooking Method:</u> same as (a) above.

(d) Air gathering with blood: pain; full feeling in the chest; feel cold and hot like "malaria;" does not like to drink or eat; liable to forget; may go into a coma or go crazy.

<u>Formula of herbs:</u> Smash 50 pieces of peach kernel to powder, cinnamon twig (120 grams), Rheum Officinale Baill (160 grams), Natrii Sulfas (80 grams), and liquorice (80 grams).

<u>Cooking Method:</u> Cook three pints of water to a boil with the peach kernels, officinale, and liquorice over a low fire for 40 minutes. Discard the sediment. Add the cinnamon twig for 10 minutes to dissolve. Discard the sediment again, then put in Natrii Sulfas for three minutes to dissolve. There is about one pint of herbal tea remaining. Drink one third of that every eight hours.

(e) Air gathering: full feeling in the chest and <u>belly</u>, and even into the <u>organs</u>; all the ribs are painful; tongue turns white; pulse is obvious but weak; annoyed and impatient. This situation is very dangerous. People can still try (a), then (c), then (d).

(B) Gathering in chest but not painful: (to omit, because that was not deemed as mesothelioma by the doctors.)

What is ironic is that there are a lot of lawsuits about "Mesothelioma caused by Asbestos," but no doctors, lawyers, and judges know the real truth, and no patients got cured. Also, no mass asbestos was found in the patient's body.

The case of the author's patient was in Boston. Her problem of Mesothelioma was solved by the author overnight with (b) formula. But that night, the patient called the author gladly and to say that she appreciated the author's help. However, she still had a problem: she felt a kind of hard dish feeling surrounding her chest. (Later on, the author found out that she had water liquid in her chest, but that is, another symptom of LUPUS that should be treated with formula (a) or (c).) That night was before Thanksgiving. I thought that could be left for her doctors to find so the doctors could be surprised about her "mesothelioma" disappearing. It turned out that on Thanksgiving, her chest blew up again. (This should have been treated with formula (d) above. It was because the bad air and water mixed and created mesothelioma again.) And she was in a coma. So, that day, the patient's husband sent her to the emergency room and she died there.

Beware: Natrii sulfas and kansui are toxic and are prohibited to be used by the FDA, but they really work for this kind of situation, as long as there was not an overdose and it was made the proper way. They save lives. The author believes the legislators and the FDA should change the laws without hesitation.

(C) Mulberry to Treat High Cholesterol and Cured It Overnight

One of the author's friends liked to steal the author's Chinese medical concepts, so he used to hang around the author's office. One day he stopped by and told the author that yesterday he found his backyard full of big houseflies. Then he found that the big tree in his backyard was full of mulberries that were so sweet and attracted all the flies. He picked a full liter container and ate them all that evening, without eating dinner. That night, he started to run to the toilet, almost every hour, but it was not diarrhea.

The next day he woke up and felt that his sight was so clear and bright, not blurred like before. Also, he felt his hands and legs were very much flexible. When I heard that, I wanted him to check his blood right away. He did.

One week later, he stopped by again. He said that his "cholesterol" had dropped to normal. Before this, his cholesterol had been very high and at a critical point, even though he had strong dose of medicine. His doctor had advice him to be very careful.

The author tried to get his blood panel report from North Carolina, but could not get it. Anyhow, this is a tip the author gives to readers. If it does not work, you can deem the author as a liar. The author wondered: is it suitable for a diabetic patient? Because the mulberry is very sweet.

(D) Herbal Treatment for Rheumatism and Arthritis

<u>DOCUMENT 1</u>

Mark Hertel
319 E 14th St, Apt 3B
New York, NY 10003
Telephone: 917-841-9433
mah2115@columbia.edu

20 March 2008
To Whom It May Concern:
I was recently treated using Chinese herbal preparations by Dr. Ming Guo Cho for acute and debilitating pain in a large area of the left side of my neck. I am very grateful to Dr. Cho for his services, which rapidly and completely cured my condition, leaving no side effects.

I first began to notice discomfort in my neck on the evening of Saturday, 8 March 2008, after I had spent considerable time during the day in Queens walking outdoors in the cold, wind and rain to attend several meetings in different locations. I was wearing a heavy coat, but it was not waterproof, and got soaked in the ice-cold rain, chilling me and dragging heavily on my neck and shoulders.

On Sunday, 9 March 2008, there was noticeable, but manageable discomfort in the left side of my neck. I awoke on the morning of Monday, 10 March 2008, with pain in a large area of the left side of my neck, which was so acute that I could only move my left arm with great difficulty. The slightest touch in the area was unbearable and even to lie down or get out of bed was excruciating. On the morning of Tuesday, 11 March 2008, the pain had grown worse, and I began to treat it using a cream whose active ingredient is the herb arnica. That cream gave noticeable temporary relief. When the pain persisted on Wednesday, 12 March 2008, I sought the advice of a few friends, one of whom recommended Dr. Cho to me. The pain persisted, and I was able to visit Dr. Cho on Friday, 14 March 2008.

Dr. Cho and I talked for a few minutes about my condition and about the theory of Chinese medicine and how Dr. Cho planned to apply it to my case. He prepared a paste made of herbs, which he vigorously rubbed on a wide area of the skin of the back of my neck, as well as on the backs of my hands. He also sprinkled some dry herbs onto the paste. He placed hot, moist padding, which he periodically reheated, on the herbal mixtures on my neck and hands. After about two hours of this treatment, I experienced a dramatic decrease in the pain, though some pain remained.

The level of pain remained steady, and I returned to Dr. Cho on Sunday, 16 March 2008, when he gave me certain quantities of the herbs Ephcdrac, cinnamon twigs, licorice, and almond. He directed me to boil the Ephedrac in a quart of water and simmer it for 50 minutes before adding the other dry ingredients and letting them simmer for another 50 minutes. Then at bedtime I was to drink 1/3 of the remaining liquid (about a pint) and drink the other 1/3 about three hours later. The next morning I was to drink the last 1/3.

I followed Dr. Cho's instructions closely. After drinking the first dose of the broth, I was unable to sleep, as my heart immediately began to beat much faster than normal, and with great force, my limbs trembled noticeably, I experienced a sensation of dryness and heat throughout my body, and my thoughts seemed to race. I felt weak, and unable to focus mentally, but the pain in my neck was virtually gone within an hour or two, and I rested in bed, awake. About three hours after going to bed, I rose to drink the second dozes of the broth. It was very bitter, and a little nauseating, so I had to drink it slowly. I continued to feel weak, shaky, and slightly feverish throughout the day. I had virtually no appetite and ate very little and drank only a few cups of water. By the morning of Tuesday, 18 March 2008 the insomnia, exhaustion, and fever were gone and I was able to resume all normal activities, including physical exercise and my corporate law practice at a large Manhattan firm. The pain in my neck was completely cured. It has not returned to any extent since I completed the treatment.

Dr. Cho's treatment brought about a rapid and complete cure of my condition. It also opened my eyes to the profound healing power of Chinese medicine. The great benefits attainable through the use of herbs should be available to the public. Qualified practioners like Dr. Cho, who are knowledgeable, responsible, and concerned about the public health and the well-being of their clients, should be free to practice their remarkably effective healing art.

Sincerely,
Mark Hertel

(E) Unnecessary Lawsuit for the Painkiller due to their Side Effects (not True)

DOCUMENT 2

December 15, 2008

To:
Mr. Jeffrey B. Kindler
CEO, Pfizer, Inc.
235 E. 42nd St.
New York, NY 10017
212-733-2323

From:
Mr. Mingguo Cho
Mingguo Alternative Healing Information Center, Inc.
63 E. Broadway, #2C
New York, NY 10002
917-406-8270
212-267-6066

Subject:
(1…) It is not necessary to pay the settlement of $884 million for the lawsuit regarding Pfizer's product Bextra, because it is ultimately not Bextra's responsibility.
(2…) Bextra belongs back on the market.

Dear Mr. Kindler,

According to the research I have conducted over the years, I have found that all pain comes from what the ancient Chinese medical books term the 'elements': for instance, Lupus is caused by the fever element (or heat); Arthritis and Fibromyalgia are caused by the wind element; Rheumatoid and Leukemia are caused by the chill element; toxins are caused by chemicals and bacteria that accumulate with the presence of fever, wind, and/or moisture. Rheumatoid is caused by moisture; and blood clots are caused by dryness.

Chinese (Oriental) medicine has different herbs to treat and cure the illnesses that arise due to different elements. It is fundamentally different from Western medicine, which merely disables the alarm, which comes in the form of pain. For example, the use of Bextra treats illness by removing pain itself—by blocking the enzyme COX-2. While this is very efficient for treating pain, the elements that actually cause the pain (what ancient Chinese medical literature refers to as "wind," "fever," "chill," "toxin," "dryness," "moisture," etc.) remain in the body.

Because it eliminates the sensation of pain, Bextra encourages patients to get back to life as usual, thinking the problem cured. In truth, the patient should be resting, as he or she would be if the pain were consciously felt. Pain is simply nature's way of alarming the patient so that he or she might get the treatment that would remove the element that is the source of the illness, not simply the pain (which is Bextra's function): pain is merely one symptom of a much larger problem that is not within Bextra's scope.

This is where Chinese herbal medicine can help. [Please see

the file enclosed.]

The patient (who is a lawyer), whose letter is enclosed, suffered from arthritic pain (caused by wind) and rheumatoid (caused by moisture and chill).

The patient had aches and pains that migrated from his neck to his arms, as is characteristic of pain caused by the wind element. If left unaddressed, this element can eventually cause heart attacks, strokes, and the Steven Johnson Syndrome. Toxic Epidermal Necrolysis may also result from the toxins created by a combination of wind, fever, and moisture. Blood clots can also form because the patient's blood can become overly dry—that may be due to the Lupus (fever) or wind in the blood, heart, or spleen.

In other words, even without Bextra, these problems (side effects) will eventually happen within the patient's systems (with wind, fever, moisture or toxin) sooner or later. Please note that I have the herbal medicine to treat and cure blood clots too.

So overall, of the following side effects to Bextra: (1) stroke, (2) heart attack, (3) blood clots, (4) Steven Johnson syndrome, (5) Toxic Epidermal Nacrolysis, (6) stomach bleeding, and (7) death, only (6) stomach bleeding is a genuine side effect of Bextra, because of its relation to the enzyme's inhibitor, that is, a large amount of live enzymes were produced from the stomach. None of the other side effects have anything to do with Bextra.

Moreover, if all the foregoing effects were truly from Bextra, then every patient who is taking Bextra should get these side effects, but not everyone does—only the patients with wind. If without this knowledge doctors remove Bextra from the market, such an action will leave many patients suffering pain without any recourse toward the right treatment for their illness. It is also unfair to Pfizer, Inc.

Please find enclosed my case reports about Lupus, Hepatitis B, and Fibroid. Although I have not graduated from medical school and lack a Ph.D., I have a high level of understanding, research, and experience with ancient Chinese medical wisdom that can do what today's western doctors cannot— that is, cure the incurable diseases. This paper's report should be the evidence: I believe I am more qualified than any other doctor to discuss this case.

Sincerely yours,
Mingguo Cho.

Author's Comments

(1...) Society is confused. (Includes: patients, doctors, pharmaceutical companies, lawyers, and government.) Wrong accusations and wrong judgment.—Pfizer's lawsuit of their product "Bextra." If the accusations and judgment were correct, then either that proved the FDA's three phases law were inadequate as what I discovered and said or the drug company had some kind of deal with the FDA. Otherwise, is that medicine "Bextra" passed through all kinds of tests, how come they did not find the side effects? Is that conspiracy, so they chose to settle? The answer is, I am right: (a) Three Phases Law was inadequate and (b) the medical industry doesn't know that, beyond the pain, there are some kinds of "elements" (real causes) that need to be removed. (Most of these illnesses and treatment mentioned are mentioned in the Chinese medical book.)

(2...) How was a young lawyer cured by me? He had pain (with wind and moist) in first stage—usually begins from Meridian of the urine bladder. If not cured, then it will go deeper and deeper to the other Meridians. (Total there is 16 Meridians in the Qi's anatomy—these are not mentioned in western medical books, but only in the Chinese medical book.) The herbal formula and this disease along with its causes are on page 26 of the Chinese medical book.

The author has more patients with other diseases, but because of the short medical evidence, the author does not want to list them all here.

The author knows that many medical professionals will say, "You only have a few cases. That does not count in the medical industry."

The author's rebuttal is: If I was a licensed pro through years of experimenting with one disease and then I found a cure, I would be considered great. Now, without any medical background, not even as a nurse or acupuncturist, I can cure LUPUS within three months even without seeing each other and have found cures for other diseases such as mesothelioma without any experiments. My great accomplishments are not me, but based on the Chinese medical books. Why do our medical professionals with all kinds of authority and privilege ignore our ancestors' valuable experience? Is that prejudice and discrimination? Should the government require them to study these ancient remedies? What the professionals find could save millions of lives.

Not only have I cured incurable diseases with proof using herbal formulas listed clearly in books—but I've also found the reasons why the western medical industry could not—because the medicines were all based on laboratory testing. And all those tests were focused on the dead tissue instead of the patients' body conditions, such as wind, chills, heat, moisture, dryness, toxins, Qi (shortage or idle, clogged). That kind of ignorance leaves the causes of almost all diseases unknown. That is what the author has been trying to advise and teach the medical industry professionals and the public, including patients. The information in this book can have positive outcomes for government and the insurance industry. The author is glad to show his progress despite the barriers.

This is the author's first book which explains his starting point. Some people still want to question: how come no other Chinese doctor could do what the author has done. For the typical example, everyone goes to a Chinese herbal doctor who is experienced and licensed. That doctor will take the patient's pulse and, according to the pulse, explain how the patient's inners are not balanced in Yin and Yang, but let the author point out clearly that all of their methods of taking pulse readings are wrong. Should the author say that all of them are liars? Yes. But can we blame them? No. Just everybody has been too busy making a living. Nobody would go to study and check the fundamental theories. So, even they were taught wrong. Unfortunately, nobody will go to study more from the foundation to find the truth.

Is that the same as the western medical industry: thousands of doctors and pharmacists who care about why there is no cure for most diseases? How come most of their causes were unknown? Why can a layman like the author do this in a short amount of time and with all kinds of barriers while the professionals could not do this for a century?

Engineers know that there are all kinds of causes for the mechanical, electrical, and chemical problems that happen in our devices. Is it ironic to say that doctors know where life comes from in evolution, but they do not know where diseases come from.

The proper way to take the pulse to find the diagnosis which is "Three Fingers Zen" from the book (See illustration below):

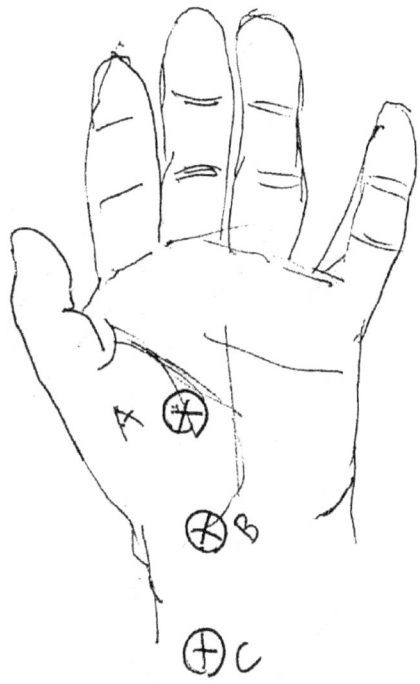

Figure 8

A point: To check upper chest, such as heart and lungs.
B point: To check lower chest, such as stomach, spleen, and liver.
C point: To check kidney, intestines.
Also, the left hand is different from the right hand.

Almost all the Chinese doctors are taking the pulse similar to the western doctors by concentrating only on point C. Western doctors are taking the pulse just to measure the count of heart beats. If the Chinese doctors are taking the pulse only at point C, most diagnoses have to do with abdominal problems. Anything the doctor says about the heart, or liver should be considered lies or a guess. But they only wondered so that does not seem accurate. However, there is nobody willing to find the truth.

For example, see below:

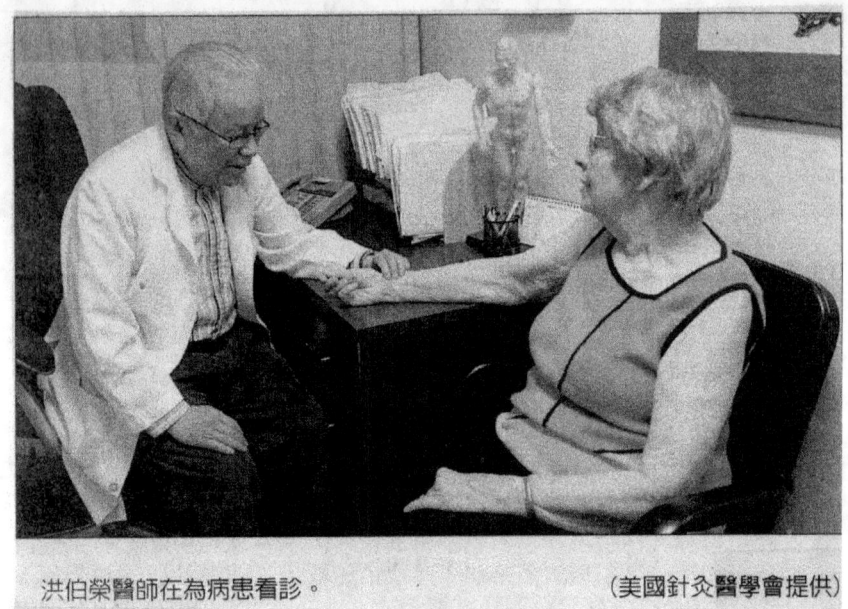

洪伯榮醫師在為病患看診。　　　　　　　　　（美國針灸醫學會提供）

Figure 9

This is Professor David P.J. Hung, O.M.D., Ph.D. He is a great acupuncture doctor. Through his effort and leadership he helped acupuncture to be accepted and legalized so the treatment and malpractice of acupuncture could be covered by insurance. He has been honored to be named the lifelong Chairman of the American Acupuncture Association (December 31, 2013). In this photo, we can see even he is taking the pulse for diagnosis the wrong way. Then should I mention any more about his students? Members? Should we blame them? Just like when I mentioned Newton was wrong: "There is no universal gravity. The so called gravity is from another cause." Whom do you believe? Whom should we blame? Does not your teacher say so? But the author will prove it is wrong in another book.

CHAPTER 13

FUNCTIONS AND UTILIZATION OF QI GONG

Twenty-five years ago, the author finished this draft. It became a joke with his friends and upset the author a little while. Somehow, he had lost this chapter without knowing it. Thanks to God, after all these years with more divisions of Qi Gong and the development of the Internet, it was easier to write this chapter. Also, the reader could check the information on the Internet.

In the contemporary world, there are a few misunderstanding about QiGong:

1...Scientists and governments said it is nonsense or witchcraft: Especially 120 years ago: the old China (Qing-Dynasty) thought they could fight the cannons and rifles of western countries with Qi Gong power, which resulted in eight countries invading China and dividing the country into separate occupations. From then on, Qi Gong became a kind of joke.

2...Religious people, mostly Christians, thought Qi-Gong was evil, due to the Bible's instruction in Isaiah 8:19-20: But people will tell you to ask for messages from fortunetellers and mediums, who chirp and mutter. They will say, 'After all, people should ask for messages from spirits and consult the dead on behalf of the living.' You are to answer them, 'Listen to what the Lord is teaching you. Don't listen to mediums; what they tell you will do you no good.'

But is the prophet not the medium after all?.

Because of the previous two reasons, for a hundred years almost no scientist was willing to waste time to practice, study, and measure Qi Gong.

And those teaching the Qi-Gong or yoga usually only emphasized meditation—to calm the mind, reduce stress, and stretch the tendons, so the body could become more flexible and not stiff.

Besides these, if trying to say more, may cause the unnecessary confusion or rejection, because most of the teachers even cannot explain it in scientific ways and with evidence.

Therefore, in this chapter, the author is willing to analyze it according to his watching, learning, engineer's point of view. In the previous chapters, the author has already simplified Qi-Gong as: accumulate energy (Qi) – store energy –applying energy.

A…Timing:

(a) Take one hundred days to build the foundation. At least practice one hour in the morning, one hour in the evening, then he can feel the energy flow in the body along the meridian. Also, feel the energy gathering below the belly button. (Ni-Chong Qi Gong by San-Chu Wu)

(b)…Take three years to reach the general completion, or at least 4 hours a day in meditation. Up to this level, the person does not need eyeglasses, and the body is full of energy so the outlook will be the same as a young man, and the gray hair will return to its original color. And if through the master's instruction, he will be able to heal himself with the inner power and also able to heal other people with his hand, but without body contact (remote healing: about 1-10 feet away) (Nei-Ging One Finger Zen by Ah-Sue Chue)

(c)…Take ten years to reach the great completion: During these seven years (after general completion), the person's third eye will be opened, and year by year, what he can see and feel in the spiritual world will be different. It turned out that in Buddhism (India) that

Buddha said, "Talk is prohibited." And in Chinese Taoism also has the same advice, "Heavenly secret should not be disclosed."

Both great religious leaders seem to be talking about the same thing that everything going to happen in the future are prearranged by a great God, although they (Qigong practitioner) through training could see a little bit of that, but since the greatest did not give permission, so silence was necessary. And one very interesting example is: the author had heard from one good fortuneteller that, since heavenly secrets (God's will about what is going to happen in the world) should not be disclosed, but some time because of sympathy or personal need, the fortuneteller will disclose it to people. So, the fortuneteller before they follow the master to learn, they had to swear to God that for his whole life he must choose one of his future as follows: poor, or physical defect, or no children. How serious it is. Of course, four hours of meditation, besides the eight hours of sleeping, every day is still necessary for ten years, but fortunetellers have their special ways to reach the spirits. Some of them do not even need meditation at all. Elisha got power from Elijah is an example. (II Kings 2)

B…Talking about function and utilization of Qi Gong, instead of just saying, the author would rather indicate a few typical samples from the Internet so readers can go to check for more details and to understand that there is proof for what the author said.

a…Falun Da Fa

This faction is new (about 40 years) and most well developed: students already number about a hundred million.

i…The grandmaster: Mr. Lee, Hong-Jhi had his third eye opened. He also teaches how to do this and what happened in his book, *Fa Lun Gong*.

ii…It is free to learn. (Books and DVD not included.)

iii…Mostly, they teach not only Qi Gong, but also the philosophy of Universe.

iv…Many of their disciples are witnesses of the miracle of their Qi Gong – Falun Gong.

Author's comment: Since they already became a faction of religion, most of the witnesses seem to emphasize the miracle instead of how the healing happened. But the Master, who is now almost seventy, looks like forty or less. Also, his book *Falun Da Fa* has details about how he opened his third eye.

Also, one thing very interesting is when the third eye open: what he can see is like watching TV. And there are news updates, along with some fiction that may be from somebody's idea or imagination. That's difficult to be separated. Maybe that is what God does not want us to ask mediums. I Kings 13: One prophet was fooled by another old prophet, disobeyed God, ate and drank, and was then killed by a lion, which is a good example.

b...Inner power one finger Zen (Nei Jing Yi Zhi Chan). It was established by a Shaolin monk Chie, Ah Suie (1919-1982). His disciples number about thirty, while his students number about three million.

i...He is the one who had a scientific record with the Chinese government's National Science Committee in 1982.

ii...One of his disciples, Master Wang, Zue Ting, is the author's teacher. He can use his hand without touching to push a few people about ten feet away (or three meters) and pull them to walk at the same time. The most amazing is to exercise a paralysis patient's leg by bending and stretching it many times remotely with his mind. Of course, he does this barehanded to give energy is their expertise, so "to heal with Qi-gong by Master" can be represented by this faction.

iii...The practice and training is divided by three steps:

1...Meditation with standing form.

2...Ten postures' exercise to practice giving out interior energy, and cover the patient's body's exterior so the patient will be influenced by the master.

3...After a little while, the patient's body will absorb the energy from the master so the disease can be healed.

Author's comment: Since to heal is using the master's own energy, so the master usually gets weaker after a treatment, unless he used one hand to absorb energy from the Universe and one hand to treat the patient, exactly like jumping a battery with the engine running or not that will make a difference. To supplement the master's own energy, he needs to drink ginseng tea or meditate four hours again is absolutely necessary. Otherwise, the grand master could have only lived 62 years, as the typical example to be understood.

The Prophet Elisha was sick with a fatal disease and died early (II Kings 13:14). He could cure the dead from death, but not himself. That is the same reason.

Also, that is the reason Falun Da Fa are emphasizing to practice yourself instead of being treated by the grand master. It is also mentioned that to treat a patient is to violate God's will—sounds like God helps those who help themselves.

c…"Ying Diau Gong" from Taoism

This faction was established by Master Tu, and also interviewed by the TV Discovery Channel.

i…It is focused on the penis and testicles to gradually lift from 2 lbs to 300 lbs.

ii…That practice can cure "prostate swollen" within one week. Also, it can enhance a man's sexual ability, obviously, and let them feel energized.

iii…This practice is very practical to see your improvement as you add weights.

Author's comment: A long time ago, the author already knew this kind of Qi-gong. However, because subconsciously he deemed this as evil, he never paid attention to it. The author believes that many people think the same, so there are not too many students of this faction. Another reason, the fees are not cheap, about two thousand U.S. dollars.

Later on through a friend's introduction, a student of this faction, Mr. Lee who is now a master, discussed Qi Gong with the author. They had an interesting exchange of information. This Mr. Lee had reached the level of lifting 200 lbs by his penis, but he is about 5'8" and skinny. The author was sparked by the idea: how can a penis—without bone and muscle—lift 200 lbs only by Qi (energy), just like a compressor can lift something heavy. This force must be great and could be measured. Also, if the author could use this force to apply on his knowledge about Qi-gong, then many functions could be more visible. So, the author decided to learn about this in the future. To learn this Qi Gong, it was necessary to have enough rest and to sleep deeply or there would obviously be injury.

Another important concept is to increase the Qi (life energy) to deliver to the testicles. That will stimulate the man's hormone and that will make people younger for sure.

d…"Ni-Zhong Qi-gong" by Master Wu, San Chu in Taiwan. This faction was established by Master Wu.

i…The technique teaches people how to build the foundation of Qigong within one hundred days.

ii…After 100 days, the energy will be sensed to pass through 12 major meridians and four vessels. The student's body will shake back and forth or swing around or jump up and down along the Qi's flowing in the different meridians.

iii…The student will feel that the movement is not because of the muscles function, but Qi's (energy) power.

iv…From the movement, the student will feel much energy he has—the more the energy the more the movement.

Author's comment: This is a very easy and practical way to know Qigong. The author recommends this for the beginners as well as for doctors, patients or anyone who questions Qigong. It is good because the person only needs to take one hour a day to practice and do it for 30 days. The feeling of "Qi" will then become very clear that nobody can deny it.

e…Talking about utilization of Qi-gong. Besides the healing and spiritual training, another important way is for the martial arts. Many people have learned about Tai-Chi Chuan. Two other famous factions are Pa-Kua Palm (Ba Gua Zhang) and Syn-Yi Chuan. All these three factions readers can find on the Internet.

The author has to correct a misunderstanding by the public: their motions are very slow. Therefore, these types of martial arts are only for health purposes, but not for real fighting.

If I mention some famous masters of these functions, such as Cheng, Mahn-Qing (Tai-Chi); Wang, Siang-Zai (Syn-Yi Chuan); and Sun, Lu-Tang (Pa-Kua Palm), people may have no feelings. They may like to make the challenge: why didn't they come in the ring to fight for money and glory? So far, the most famous Kung-fu fighter is Bruce Lee, but he is not a Qi-gong boxer. His fighting philosophy is "Speedy." But, if I mention a boxing champion—Mike Tyson, people may laugh.

Yes, he did not learn Qi-gong at all, not even any kung fu, but he was born to be a fighter. He gained his title at age 18 after only two years of training. Since he was adopted by Mr. Jacob, his lifestyle has been very simple, much like a Shao-Lin monk in training. He had no girlfriend. That was the key. So his ability to become a champion was not through any famous coach, but through his loving, caring adopted father. Then, he lost his title just because he got married and lost Mr. Jacob (out of control). Now, let us analyze this special case:

1…If Tyson had been trained by a good coach, he could have rehired the coach and regained his title. But, there was no such coach.

2…If he had a training with a good coach, it would take at least three years to gain a title, such as Ali and Sugar Ray had done. And he wouldn't have lost his ability.

3…Review of Tyson's tournaments:

a…His fighting always finished within one or two rounds.

b…His fighting not as complicated as the fighting shown in the *Rocky* movie, but just like Magnetic Bar: within a very short distance, whenever the opponent punched, his head could just swing away smoothly, exactly the same as when you push a magnetic bar's positive to another magnetic bar's positive. Before it reaches, the bar will swing away. Also, his eyes would stare at the opponent all the time (not like other boxer's with heads bowed down to avoid punches, so the eyes were looking at the ground). He could get the best opportunity and location to launch his fist. Because the opponent had already gone too far to return, they could never dodge to get away.

c…This kind of magnetic feeling is what Qi-gong martial arts tried to teach in order to gain this ability. Some students have said some masters could fight even with his back to the attacker. This kind of utilization also can be found in Japanese Samurai books. The most famous one is Yagyu Sessyusai, who was the creator of Ninja and also the head of the body guard of Sho-Gun; he executed his duty without carrying a sword, meaning he could defeat any samurai with his bare hands. Even the famous Samurai Myamoto Musashi admitted he is not as good as the Master Yagyu.

d…After Tyson got married, because of his sex life, his volume of sperm should be reduced, unless somebody taught him to avoid having sex three months before a fight.

e…So, when he fought Evander Holyfield, Tyson did not know he already lost his sensitive ability. Therefore, after a few punches by Holyfield, Tyson felt scared and mad, because he never had been punched like that. But this time, it seemed any punch would hit him, so he struggled and bit off a portion of Holyfield's ear.

f…Of course, after this, he could never regain his title back. Because he did not know why. Neither did his new manager, Mr. Don King. This is exactly the same as Samson in the Bible (Judges 12-16) who got super strength and lost it because his hair stored and released "Qi" (energy).

g…The author tried to tell Tyson. Tyson seemed too shy. Long after writing Tyson a letter, he called back without identifying himself and asked the author, "Are you a coach?" I said "no." Then he hung up without any more communication,

h…So, people, including Tyson himself, wondered why he could not do as Ali could, who lost his title and regained it back. Although Tyson was born to be a fighter, and did not gain his title through special training.

i…Tyson should be able to get this ability back before he is 50 years old, as long as he knows the concept of "Qi." He should not have any sex six months prior to a fight, and have regular boxing training. These should be enough for him to win. Make sure in training he can dodge away from the trainer's punches automatically. Then, he could gain his title back for sure.

CHAPTER 14

QUESTIONS AND ANSWERS

Question #1 AIDS is known to be caused by a virus. It has been photographed and identified. Magnetic fields may not explain a virus-caused disease.

Answer...Doctors say that AIDS is caused by a virus, which they think came from the ape family. That has been misleading in the same way doctors said mesothelioma came from asbestos. The author has proved they are not related at all:

...(1)...never has anyone gotten the AIDS virus from being bitten by a gorilla

...(2)...never has anyone had intercourse with a gorilla

...(3)...the AIDS virus was originally created from gay men who were the receivers (female roles), but not the ones who acted in the male role. That created the excuse that AIDS did not come from homosexuality.

...(4)...the gay man receiver, after a certain period (depending on the frequency of anal intercourse) would have the AIDS symptoms first, but without the virus. So, doctors won't see him as an AIDS patient at this stage until later on. The virus started to be produced. Then, this patient is put on the AIDS patient list.

This is similar to the LUPUS patient. The patient had a fever first, and then had his ds DNA figure increased. The antigen was created by organs under certain conditions.

So as the leukemia (blood cancer): when the kidney's temperature was brought up, the WBC (white blood cell) amount would be dropped. It is happening with the author's LUPUS patients all the time.

…(5)…What the author focuses on is the original cause. And this concept can be applied to all kinds of flu—environmental conditions caused the flu first and then the flu viruses were produced when the weather changed. After a little while, the flu should disappear as well as the virus.

Question #2 Anal intercourse has been not only one source of the AIDS transmission. AIDS can also be transmitted between heterosexual couples, one of whom has the AIDS virus.

Answer: Again, what the author emphasized is the condom (rubber) cannot block the magnetic influence during anal intercourse to damage the sphere field which then produces the virus.

Question #3 Vaginal intercourse or oral sex has nothing to do with magnetic fields?

Answer: Vaginal intercourse is actually good for the magnetic field. The Chinese call that Yin-Yang Harmony (that means positive and negative balance) – special when the penis goes into the uterus.

Oral sex has nothing to do with the magnetic field.

Overall, it can be said: the points get involved are the points of Qi's (life energy) concentration: in yoga, the illustration below shows there are five points on the center line of the human body: (1) top of head is the center of hair whirl, (2) Heavenly Eye: one inch up between the two eyes, (3) Upper Dan-tien: between the two nipples; (4) Middle Dan-tien – the sphere field, about the position of the uterus; and (5) Lower Dan-tien, about the position of the prostate, Also called "Huey Ying" this is the point that can be influenced by anal intercourse.

ILLUSTRATION – FIVE BODY POINTS

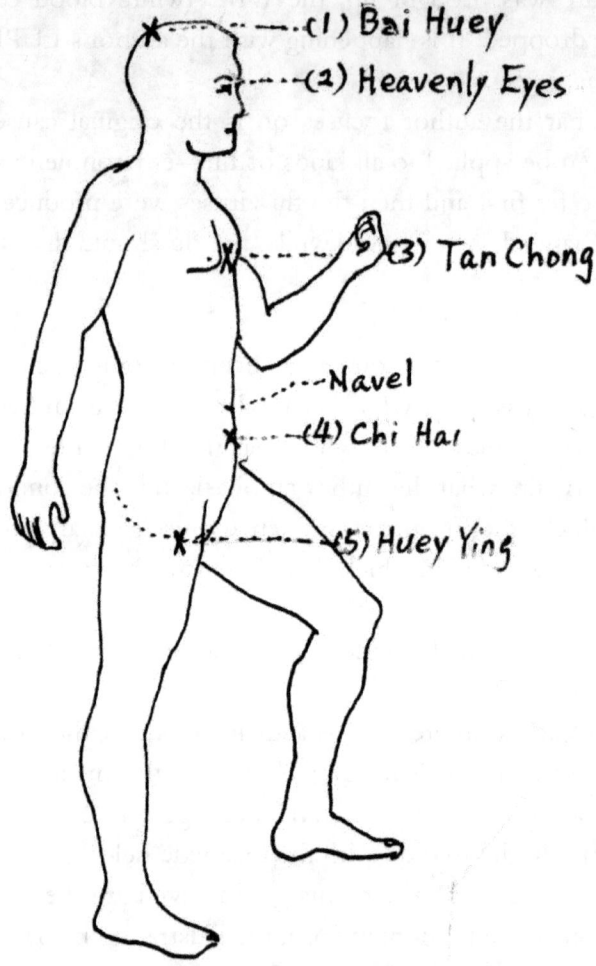

(1) Bai Huey
(2) Heavenly Eyes
(3) Tan Chong
Navel
(4) Chi Hai
(5) Huey Ying

Figure 10

Question #4 Condoms cannot protect the magnetic field? There is no scientific evidence about the human body's magnetic fields.

Answer: Condoms (rubber) cannot protect the magnetic field. There is no scientific evidence about the human body's magnetic field is not true. Most people's magnetic field is not strong enough for them to be aware of it. The reader must check the Internet: some people can use their bodies to attract a metal knife, spoon, and so on. See the illustration below.

ILLUSTRATION – HUMAN MAGNETS

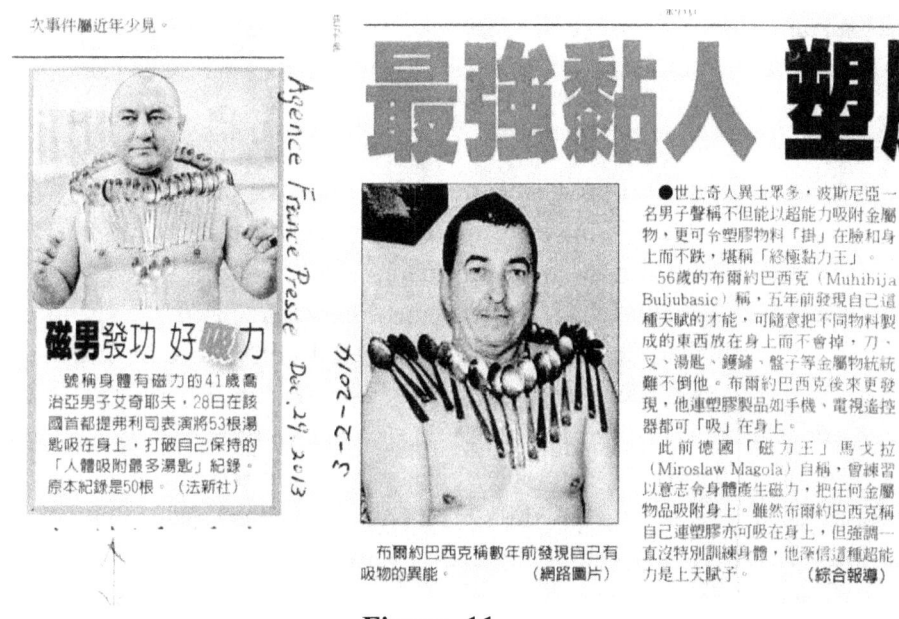

Figure 11

Magnetic Man's Powerful Attraction

(Photo on the left) The 41 year old man, Igelyeve from Georgia, claims his body has magnetic force (December 28, 2013) at the country's capital, Tbilisi. He shows that his body can attract 53 soup spoons. That breaks his own record of 50 pieces of spoons—"The most pieces of soup spoons ever attracted by the human body." Original news from Agence France Presse (December 29, 2013).

(Photo on the right) The 56 year old, Muhibija Buljubasic, from Persia (Iran) found that he has ESP to attract many things made from different materials, besides metal, such as cell phones, TV remote controls. Before, Germany's "King of Attractions" Miroslaw Magola claimed that through training he could use his will to attract metal things. But Buljubasic emphasized that he did not get any training. He sees the attraction as a kind of gift.

Also, the author has learned from two types of Qi-Gong: "Inner Strength One Finger Zen" and "Tai Gi Five Elements Gong." Both the masters can use their magnetic force to pull and push people remotely. They did come to New York City to teach. They also had many disciples in the world.

Question #5 There is too much emphasis on the unproven magnetic fields. If they are proven, list the scientific research that proves the importance of the magnetic fields.
Answer: Twenty-five years ago when the author tried to explain Qi Gong with the scientific means, he was still not mature in Qi Gong. He tried as much as possible to use the word people could understand. However, the Qi Gong or Yoga actually was well known by oriental people, especially those who knew the ancient Chinese medical textbooks. And the Qi (energy and sphere field, Dan-Tien) are clearly mentioned and taught to lead and gather the Qi in the Sphere Field, similar as a battery, but not electricity. And the force is there, so the author could only use the magnetic force to describe it. In the end, he was pretty close, but still had a difference, such as magnetic force only happens between iron and a magnetic stone. But Qi it seems can apply to all living beings. (To attract metal, only a very few special people can do this and, so far, he has never heard of any Qi Gong master who can do this.) The author wonders that the magnet is similar like light that can be separated as red, orange, and purple as seen in a prism. But the different parts of light are still contained in the same light. Besides the visible light, there are also X-

rays and other forms of invisible light.

The "scientific research," what the author knows about is "Qi-Gong." This project was supported by research grants from Academia Sinica Taipei and Rocky Foundation. Accepted for publication in Jonas, W. et al, Ed "A Textbook for Complimented Alternative Medicine" to be published by Williams and Wilkins, 1997. The scholars are Lee, Qing-Tse, Ph.D. Professor, and Chairperson Lei, Ting, Ph.D., Visiting Scholar, Department of Psychology, Brooklyn College of the City University of New York. (Note: Dr. Qing-Tse Lee is the author's teacher.)

Question #6   Stopping anal intercourse alone cannot stop the spread of AIDS.

Answer: That is right: stopping anal intercourse alone cannot stop the spread of AIDS. However, that will stop the creation of the original VIRUS. So the amount of the patient of Type One who has symptoms, but without the VIRUS should be reduced and disappear. Also, the other types of AIDS patients will be easier under the control and with asceticism, there will be more effectively cured.

Question #7   There needs to be scientific evidence that Qi Gong helps to heal. Why is it special to someone's health? Yoga also helps to reduce stress, but no mention is made of yoga.

Answer…So far, very few doctors or scholars do this kind of research. However, if the readers check the most popular Qi-gong internet, "Fa Lun Da Far," they will find out why they have almost a billion followers.

It's not that Qi Gong is special to someone's health, but health means the person's life energy (Qi) is strong. In the Japanese greeting, someone will say, "A na ta wua, gein Qi (Original Qi) le su ga," which means "how are you?"

Reducing stress is one and the beginning of Yoga's functions. Yoga is Qi Gong. In India, it is called yoga. In China or Japan, it is called Qi Gong. Yoga is the same as Qi Gong. There are many different divisions. To focus and become expert on one special functions of yoga (Qi Gong) is the reason to divide.

Yoga's meaning is "response to Heavenly God." Chinese in Daoism said the procedure of training is:

(a) to accumulate sperm transforms to Qi
(b) to accumulate Qi transforms to spirit
(c) to refine spirit back to formless
(d) to refine formless into Dao (word or God)

So, if the reader wants to go to the library to check, he will find yoga is not only to reduce stress. But the way to find and unite with God.

Question #8   Can a machine be developed to influence the cells' magnetic fields?

Answer: The author wishes that the scientists would develop a machine to change Qi to enlarge the cells' magnetic field, but it seems impossible. If what the author suspects is true: "the smallest material is magneton (not quantum nor quark)" is correct. Then, nothing can catch magneton, same as nobody can catch photon (light), but light is filled over our living space during daytime. However, to enlarge Qi and its magnetic field, people can either practice Qi Gong or eat ginseng or both. Of course, eating ginseng is the most popular and easy way.

Question #9   It has already been suggested people can wear small magnets to help improve their health. What about this type of preventative therapy?

Answer: "To wear small magnets to help their health" is the rough idea of business, since the magnet has direction, the same direction is helpful. Reverse is not and is even harmful. So, as the preventative therapy, the person who develops this type of therapy must be very sensitive about the direction. In Chinese, many Qi Gong masters do suggest to wear jade stone maybe for that reason, though the author did not confirm. But in the Bible (Exodus 20:25), "If you make an altar of stone for me, do not build it out of cut stones, but use the stone naturally washed by water, because when you use a chisel on stones, you make them unfit for my use."

In physics, using the chisel to cut stones will create the magnetic field that will disturb the original magnetic field. However, there is an interesting question: what is God scared of? People are not afraid of it. God is scared of pork, while people enjoy eating pork.

Also, II Samuel 6:6-7, "As they came to the threshing place of Nacon, the oxen stumbled, and Uzzah reached out, and took hold of the covenant box. At once, the Lord God became angry with Uzzah and killed him because of his irreverence. Uzzah died there beside the covenant box.

People who read these verses will be shocked: the one who tried to protect God's Covenant was killed. Why was God angry and what made Uzzah deserve the death penalty? Is God nuts or absurd? Even King David could not understand. But now, if you have my concept of magnetic field, then you will realize that "Holy" means: people's magnetic field is clean. If you are not clean, then you cannot stay in God's field or say even in Heaven. You will be killed or burned. And that is the reason kosher food was emphasized. That has nothing to do with God's anger.

See Matthew 22:1-14. In verse 10, we read: "So the servants went out into the streets and gathered all the people they could find (means Christian), good and bad alike; and the wedding hall was filled with people. The king went in to look at the guests and saw a man who was not wearing wedding clothes. 'Friend, how did you get in here, without wedding clothes?' the king asked him. But the man said nothing. Then the king told the servants, 'Tie him up hand and foot, and throw him outside in the dark There he will cry and gnash his teeth.' And Jesus concluded: 'Many are invited, but few are chosen'"—wearing wedding clothes means eating kosher food.

Something more to know is why God would burn the two cities of Sodom and Gomorrah (Genesis 18). Were their children a violation too? No, but they got AIDS (unclean). Of course, all these are the author's understanding, but besides these reasons and concepts, nothing else can explain it.

Later on in Jonah 4:11, God explained it. That is the proof: "How much more then should I have pity on Nineveh, that great city. After all, it has more than 120,000 innocent children in it, as well as many animals."

When the author mentions "Bible," many will challenge that "there is no God." The universe expanded from the "Big Bang." However, in Exodus 30:34-38, the Lord said to Moses, "Take an equal part of each of the sweet spices—stacte, onycha, galbanum, and pure frankincense. Use them to make incense, mixed like perfume. Add salt to keep it pure and holy. Beat part of it into a fine powder, take it into the tent of my presence, and sprinkle it in front of the Covenant Box. Treat this incense as completely holy. DO NOT USE THE SAME FORMULA TO MAKE ANY INCENSE LIKE IT FOR YOURSELVES. TREAT IT AS A HOLY THING DEDICATED TO ME. IF ANYONE MAKES ANY LIKE IT FOR USE AS PERFUME OR EVEN TO SMELL IT, HE WILL NO LONGER BE CONSIDERED ONE OF MY PEOPLE. (Some books translate: SHOULD BE KILLED.)

Also, beware that anyone makes this perfume. He will be killed. Not by people, but by God Himself. Because nobody ever smelled it before. So, even though somebody did it, nobody will be aware that perfume is not supposed to be made. Then who could sense and make judgment on the guy? So the only one to sense it and execute this law should be God himself. Before that time, nobody knew this formula, neither did Moses. This is God's formula.

Anyone who wants to challenge this may try this. May God forgive the author to advise you to put the LORD your God to the test. He does this to help people to know "God is there."

Question #10 Is the definition of death needed?
Answer: The definition of death is very important to be needed because without that doctors or people will easily say someone is dead. No point to rescue. As a matter of fact, many cases should be

worked on and many lives should be saved, instead of giving up. See my website: Mingguo's Alternative Healing Center. (It is temporarily offline for lack of financial support.)

A few cases were downloaded to show as reference below.

Sudden Infant Death Syndrome
Drowned
Freezing to Death
Death Caused by Hanging or Strangling

SUDDEN INFANT DEATH SYNDROME

CAUSE: Babies are badly influenced by extreme weather, such as cold, heat, dryness, or suffocation and may seem to die of unexpected reasons. In reality, problems with such things as phlegm, Qi, or heat leading to the baby becoming unconscious.

TREATMENT: Before the ambulance comes, the parent should try to use the nail of the thumb to dig into the ren zhong point. The baby will usually wake up and crfy. If there is no response, then use your nail to press the hegu (L.I. 4) point. If there is still no response, then use a moxa pill and put it on the zhong chong point and burn it (moxibustion). This is the last step and it should work. If you cannot get a moxa pill during that critical time, you may use a cigarette instead.

P.S. 1…Even if the baby's heart has stopped beating for 10 hours, there is still hope; don't give up.

2…When you use a cigarette to stimulate the baby, you have to put the cigarette over the finger tip. Don't put it underneath. Otherwise, it may be too hot, which may cause other problems.

3…All doctors and Emergency Aid workers should know this method.

Quoted from *Secret Formulas for Hundred of Diseases* (P. 153)

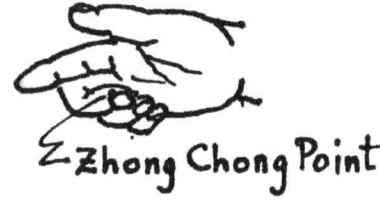
Zhong Chong Point

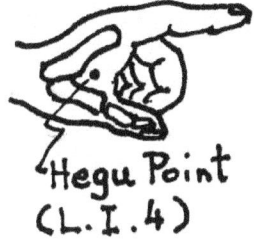
Hegu Point (L.I.4)

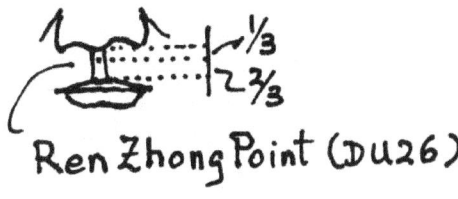
Ren Zhong Point (DU26)

Figure 12

DROWNED

TREATMENT: When a person drowns to death, as long as water is the only factor in drowning (ie: head concussion), within 10 hours (night time) to 12 hours (daytime), the patient should still be able to be rescued and cured. For a baby, maybe within 24 hours.

    I...Use charcoal ash and make a bed on the ground around 2 feet x 6 feet x 5 inches (thick).
      II...Let the cadaver lie down on the ash-bed, then cover the body with ash, including the head and feet. Within half an hour, the

water will automatically flow out from the mouth and nose. Then the patient will wake up.

   III…The time it takes to cure the patient, depends on how long the patient has died, usually no longer than one hour.

   IV…Remember "Don't try to push the chest or stomach" in case the water is stuck in a channel and cannot get out. That will cause more trouble to take out the water.

Theory: This theory is called "soil can against the water," one of the five theories of Five Elements: "Water against fire, fire against metal, metal against wood, wood against soil, soil against water." (Quote from Yi-Chong-Gin-Gian, p. 348)

Experiment: This experiment works from the house-fly to a monkey or even a pig. Mr. Mingguo Cho experimented with the house-fly. The experiment was successful.

Suggestion: All the beaches and swimming pools should have at least 12 feet of ash in buckets for emergency drowning.

FREEZING TO DEATH

CAUSE: either from cold weather or locked within a freezer.
TREATMENT: As long as the tissue cells are not broken through expanding when it is 4 degrees Celsius.

1…Within 10-12 hours, the patient should be able to be rescued.
2…Don't warm the body right away at the beginning. Otherwise, there would be no chance of recovery for the patient.
3…Prepare one gallon of warm charcoal ash.
4…Prepare one pair of socks.
5…Fill the sock with the warm ash about one fistful amount and put

it directly on top of the heart.

6…Whenever it gets cold, change to another sock of warm ash (about 10-20 minutes).

7…When the heart is getting warmer, the chi and the blood will start to circulate again and the eyes and mouth will open.

8…Start to feed with warm rice soup, barley soup, chicken broth, ginseng tea, or red wine. The Chinese books said to use rice soup and add it with the young boy's urine. (Young boy's urine is as good as ginseng.)

9…Start to massage the entire body.

Quote from Hua-Tuo *The Wander Doctor's Proprietary Nostrum* (P. 346)

DEATH CAUSED BY HANGING OR STRANGLING

CAUSE: from suicide or crime

TREATMENT: All deaths caused by hanging or strangling, as long as the spine and marrow are not disconnected within 8 hours (hung at night) to 12 hours (hung at day), can be reversed. Four persons are needed to carry out the treatment.

I.   Gently hold the cadaver and take it out of the ropes, so as not to add any more injury to the body. Place the body on a comforter or sleeping bag on the ground.

a…One person sits on the ground, holds onto the hair of the cadaver, using their legs on top of the cadaver's two shoulders, and pulls.

b…The second person pumps the heart and chest by pushing and releasing.

c…The third person massages both arms and continues to bend and pull. If the arms are already stiff, the person must bend them slowly and gradually.

d…One healthy person (his hand must be warmer than the average person's hand) massages the cadaver's abdomen.

Within one hour, the cadaver will start to breath, and open their eyes. Keep doing this motion of pulling and pushing for another 10 minutes. Then feed the patient with warm rice soup or barley soup. (Quote from Yi-Chong-Gin-Gian P. 347)

II.   Collect the following:

Goat blood 7.5 g

Rhizoma Acori Graminei 7.5 g

Folium Perillae 7.5 g

Radix Ginseng 11.25 g

Rhizoma Pinelliae (Pinellia Tuber) 11.25 g

Flos Carthami (Safflower) 3.75 g

Spina Gleditsiae (Chinese honeylocust spine) 3.75 g

Moschus (Musk) 3.75 g

Grind as a dose. Make pills, mixed with honey, as large as marbles. Save it. Mix 1 cup of rice wine to dissolve. Then, take an absorption tube to feed into the patient's throat. (Be careful not the break the glass of the tube by biting into it. After a little while, the patient should wake up. This pill works very effectively.) (Quote from P. 345.)

III.   If the patient was strangled to death, before doing the same rescue method aforesaid, we should solve the problem of the neck-artery blocking first: Just like in the game of wrestling, the key is to hit the point on the spine. Measure the point by finding the distance between the large cervical vertebra bone to the point that is the same as the patient's tip of the middle finger to the carpal bone.

Question #11…Those people working on nutrition, exercise, and reducing stress may reduce the chances of an early death, but these things are only part of the methods to prolong life. Without the concept in this book, people will never understand that old text in the Bible where some ancestors could live five hundred years or more. Nobody could do this in this century. Is the Bible fiction? No. In the Chinese medical book entitled *Emperor Huang Inner Textbook*, which is more than 3,000 years old, it also mentions in the beginning: Emperor Huang asked the doctor that he had heard about their ancestors living for hundreds of years, but why only to sixty or seventy now?

Answer: In Genesis 6:3, the Bible says, "Then the Lord said, My spirit shall not always strive with man. For that, he also is flesh: yet his days shall be an hundred and twenty years."

The answer of the doctor from the *Inner Textbook* is: Ancient people before 4,000 years ago knew the word (Dao), followed Ying and Yang, harmony with numbers, eating and drinking with control, sleeping and waking on time, never overworking, so their bodies and spirits were maintained at the full level. That is why they could enjoy their life for hundreds of years. Now today 3,000 years later, people behave the opposite way: they drank only wine, partied all the time, went to bed drunk, dried their sperm/semen with sex desires, used up all their spirit (energy), had no awareness of maintaining their level, too often lived wildly, did not care about sleeping and working off schedule. The results were that people started dying at age fifty. This was amazing that the Bible and the ancient oriental books pointed to the same fact: People can live longer than 500 years, as long as they know how. Therefore, the Bible did not lie about people living long lives.

Question #12… The lack of scientific, medical or Chinese literature supporting these ideas is completely lacking?

Answer: Again, the recharge system is there, only people do not sense it well. The most understandable case is "sleeping;" and Qi

Gong" is the concentration of "sleeping." One hour of Qi Gong practice is equal to two hours of sleeping. So some masters practice four hours Qi Gong instead of sleeping eight hours. The most famous case is the real Shao-Lin monk Master HaiDen (Sea-Lamp), who can use one finger to support himself up-side-down. He never slept, but always meditated instead. He was one of the teachers who taught movie star Jet Li.

Question #13…"The electrical system is not the loop system, but the nerve system." Blood has a loop system, but nerves in the body do not loop. Then what could the Qi's loop system be? (Can it be proven there is a Qi or that Qi is a loop?)
Answer: Actually, the electrical system is a loop. People said "no" because they neglected the "ground."

The nerves in the body seem not to loop, but as a matter of fact, they are in a loop. But because the loop is in the same nerves, they do not look like a loop.

Also, Qi's loop system exists, If people go to check the Acupuncture Illustration, they will find most acupuncture points are on the major sixteen lines (meridians). The interesting part is that all the lines seem from one end to the other end, but, if you learn Qi Gong, you will sense these lines are all connected "invisibly." Because in anatomy doctors could not find these major lines (meridians), that is why the Qi system has been neglected and ignored, even until today. Just because these lines and points are invisible, Qi is seen as the smallest material which cannot be caught by any tools. Also, it can penetrate through any material, yet fills the whole universe. The magnet is part of "Qi," similar as X-rays are part of light. And that will explain what the "gravity" really is. There is no "universal gravity," so Newton was mistaken.
This part is found by the author and will be explained in a separate book about physics.

Question #14 Is Qi more a philosophy rather than a science?

According to the author's understanding and study that he has made, the Qi and Qi Gong are the highest level of science, which can bring people from practical material to abstract, the invisible and untouchable God.

(1)… sperm → Qi → Spirit → Vanity → Dao (Word or God).

These are the levels of Qi's practicing in "Daoism." (The Chinese original religion and philosophy- exactly the same as Yoga means "meditate to respond to God."

(2)… Flesh Eyes → Heavenly Eye (third eye) → Occult Eye (propagate eyes) → Wisdom Eye (deva eyes) → Buddha's Eyes These are the levels of yoga practice (Since Chinese "Zen" and "Buddhism" are actually taught and originated from India. Shaolin Kung Fu is the typical example.)

(i)…Flesh Eyes: People's Eye became good eyesight so can get rid of eyeglasses after three years incentive practice (four hours a day at least) plus eight hours of normal sleep or sixteen hours of sleeping instead as a baby does..

(ii)…Heavenly Eye: the Third Eye opened so he can see the incidents that happened yesterday and what is going to happen tomorrow. Up to then, people will learn that everything is prearranged.

Today: "Fa Lun Gong's master, Mr. Hong-Chi, Lee can do this and he also teaches   people how to open the Third Eye. (People may check on the Internet.)

(iii)…Occult Eye (or Propagate Eye): can see the incidents that happened years before and after. That is how Jesus could tell the lady that she had five husbands and the one who lives with her now is not her husband. (John 4:16-19)

(iv)…Wisdom Eye (Deva eye): can see the incidents that happened generations before and after, such as reincarnation. (For example, Jesus said "John the Baptist is the reincarnation of Elijah, the prophet.") (Matthew 11:14)

(v)… Buddha's Eye: can see the whole picture of the spiritual world. That is how "Job" in the Bible could be described as somebody reported from a live show as an eyewitness. And actually, Jesus said nobody ever saw God Jehovah. Both stories are not contradictory.

#15 The Faraday needs a better explanation for a lay person.
Answer: Michael Faraday (1791-1867), a famous scientist, found the relation between the magnetic field, electric flow, and force. Thus, the motor and generator were developed.

See Illustration in Chapter 2
Author's Notes: Magnetic Fields

Question #16 Why do they reversal? Any benefit?
Answer: In the body's meridian, the Chinese medical textbook says, "Blood is the 'Train Car' or 'Trailer' to carry the nutrition and trash. Qi is the Head of the Train or Trailer." Without Qi, the train cannot move, even though the heart is still pumping. That is why acupuncture can stop bleeding and sensation during surgery.

Since then, we know the blood system has its direction that cannot be reversed. Also the typical diseases, such as Alzheimer's and M.S. (Multiple Sclerosis) are caused by "Qi" blocked in the meridian—this is found by the author from Chinese martial art textbook of killing by hitting acupuncture points.

Alzheimer's is caused by hitting the point of "Sen-men" (Spirit Gate), which is on Heart (mind) meridian. That is why the patient will be out of their mind. That happened most of the time when the senior patient fell and used the hand to stop the fall to the ground. M.S. is caused by hitting the point of "Fu-Ai" which is on the spleen (muscle) meridian, located on the lower chest. That will stop the energy from going into all muscles.

But except in the meridian, the Qi's flowing supposedly can be reversed, especially when the Master, using "Qi" to heal people or to change the weak patient, if he uses his own "Qi." Then the master cannot last long. Most of the time he will use his one hand to absorb

Qi from the universe and the other hand to give out "Qi" to the patient. So, he does not waste his own "Qi."

To give Qi, we will call yang (or positive). To absorb Qi, we will call yin (or negative).

Question #17   So, do we treat with drugs to kill the AIDS virus or skip the drugs? AIDS drugs have been able to keep the disease under control and the patients now live longer because of the drugs.
Answer: At this stage, the studies have said the AIDS virus can infect healthy people by blood transfusions, so the existing AIDS virus still needs drugs to treat it in order to get efficient results.

As the author's concept shows: the drugs have been able to keep the disease under control for only those people who are not gay men, but this condition cannot be proved so far, because doctors could not classify patients into five groups due to privacy concerns. These five groups are: **(1)** patients with AIDS symptoms, but without the HIV virus (Those are gay men who perform as the receiver during intercourse and women who very often used electrical sexual toys); **(2)** the patients with HIV virus, but without the AIDS symptoms (These are people infected by blood transfusions or by regular heterosexual intercourse. They are the people who are the best under control by drugs.); **(3)** For those patients who have AIDS symptoms and who also have the HIV virus, they need to be classified as **(a)** gay men (who act as women); **(b)** lesbians who have very often used electrical sex toys in the vagina; and **(c)** people who had a normal sex life and got the disease though infection. That is why the author supports the legalization of homosexual marriages and register their sexual habits. Also, the public bathrooms should be separated according to their I.D.: male, female, gay males who see men as woman, gay females who are men and act as women – lesbian men and lesbian women. Then medical doctors will find easily the theory of what the author said is true and then hopefully be able to stop and prevent the future spread of AIDS.

ADVICE: AIDS PATIENTS SHOULD BE CLASSIFIED INTO

FIVE GROUPS FOR RESEARCH.

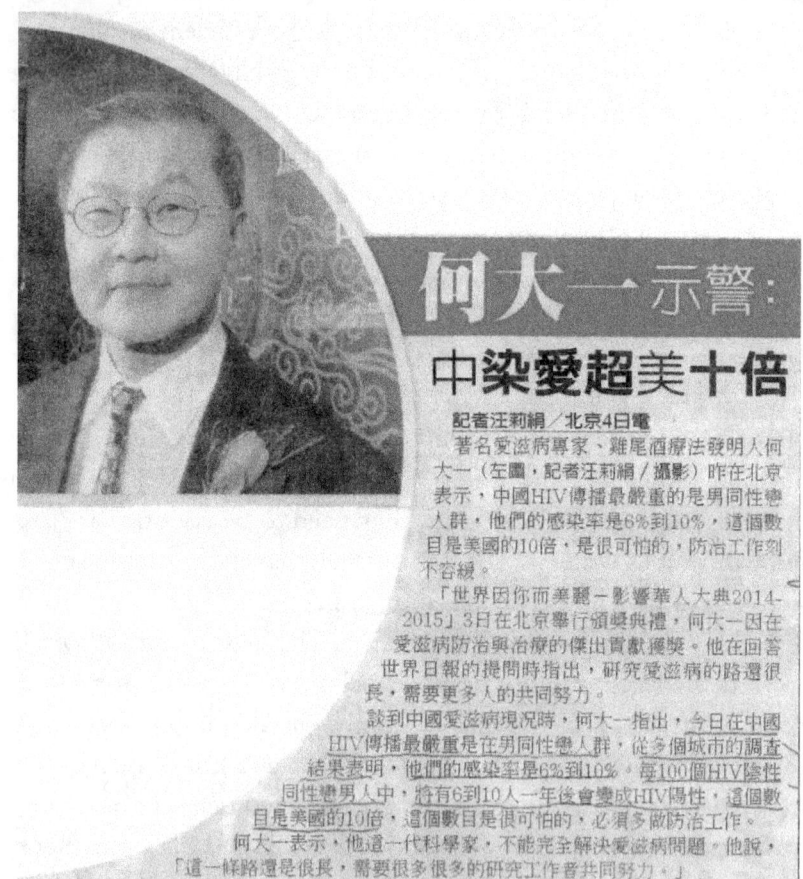

何大一示警：

中染愛超美十倍

記者汪莉絹／北京4日電

著名愛滋病專家、雞尾酒療法發明人何大一（左圖，記者汪莉絹／攝影）昨在北京表示，中國HIV傳播最嚴重的是男同性戀人群，他們的感染率是6%到10%，這個數目是美國的10倍，是很可怕的，防治工作刻不容緩。

「世界因你而美麗－影響華人大典2014-2015」3日在北京舉行頒獎典禮，何大一因在愛滋病防治與治療的傑出貢獻獲獎。他在回答世界日報的提問時指出，研究愛滋病的路還很長，需要更多人的共同努力。

談到中國愛滋病現況時，何大一指出，今日在中國HIV傳播最嚴重是在男同性戀人群，從多個城市的調查結果表明，他們的感染率是6%到10%。每100個HIV陰性同性戀男人中，將有6到10人一年後會變成HIV陽性，這個數目是美國的10倍，這個數目是很可怕的，必須多做防治工作。

何大一表示，他這一代科學家，不能完全解決愛滋病問題。他說，「這一條路還是很長，需要很多很多的研究工作者共同努力。」

Figure 13

Doctor Ho said in Bejin, China (4-4-15) that within 100 "HIV

142

SPHERE FIELDS, QI GONG AND AIDS

negative" gay men there will be 6-10 who turn "HIV positive." This number is ten times that of American gay men. This news is proof of what the author said. (*World Journal Weekly Supplement*)

Question #18 What is the relationship between Qi Gong and drugs?

Answer: As the author explained before, Qi Gong is "Life Energy" function. In this book, the author emphasizes when energy is strong enough, many diseases should disappear by themselves and vice versa. That can be understood why senior people have many more diseases than younger people.

Also, when people catch a cold (flu – virus), doctors always say: "More rest, sleep to restore the energy." In the Chinese herbal textbook, ginseng is very important, because it can give "Qi" to the human body. BUT WESTERN DRUGS MOST OF THE TIME ONLY FOCUS ON BACTERIA, VIRUSES, and ANTIGENS. THEY NEGLECT WHERE AND HOW THEY CAME IN OR HOW THEY DEVELOP FROM HUMAN TISSUE. THAT IS WHY MANY DRUGS WERE TESTED SUCCESSFULLY IN THE LABS, BUT END UP FAILING IN THE HUMAN BODY, BECAUSE THE SCIENTISTS NEGLECT THE ENVIRONMENTAL CONDITIONS. However, these drugs are very efficient to treat whatever they wanted to treat. That cannot be denied absolutely. The doctors were just confused since their drugs or operations killed the bacteria, viruses, antigen or cancer cells completely, but why were they growing back again later on?

Question #19 Are there certain herbs and foods that cooperate with Qi-gong?

Answer: Yes, ginseng is the most typical herb. However, there are different kinds of ginseng:

Korean ginseng: the strongest one, one finger large already can provide a lot of energy. If overdosed, the person will have a headache or nose bleed. But when people are in the critical point, the Korean ginseng can help a lot, such as during a baby's delivery. Sometimes, the mother will bleed and cannot stop. If she is given a slice of Korean ginseng under the tongue, that will stop the bleeding.

American ginseng: is helpful for senior people and administered as a daily supplement because it is not that strong.

Chinese ginseng (Pilose Asiabell Root): mostly used in Chinese herbal formulas (Scrophularia root).

Black ginseng: mostly used for the patients who had a fever in the organs and blood, because it will give energy, but also cool down the fever.

Sand ginseng (Adenophora root): good for lung and stomach and for those patients who feel "dry."

Red Sage Root: good for heart and liver.

Also, there are many others, such as Astragalus Root, Lucid Ganoderma, but too many to mention all their functions here.

Question #20 Absorbing the female's secretion (absorbing the female fluid is not accurate while in intercourse?):

Answer: It is true, but only most men neglect this part. In yoga or Qi Gong, there are division (or faction) specialties in this kind of method. So people can even see in India's temple, there are some pictures on the wall to teach that. But the people in good division see that as evil and prevent a discussion of that. Because through that way, the man will be stronger, but the woman will be looking old soon. The other proof is "If men would not absorb the female's fluid, then the men should not get venereal diseases through sexual contact and contract from women.

Question #21 Are there better explanations or Internet links to explain such phenomena, because some may consider these locations as fantasy of the imagination and not factual.

Answer: This is not imagination, actually in China and Taiwan, many locations are famous for these kinds of phenomena, such as cars slide up when in neutral, instead of down on the sloped street and water flows up in a stream. Rain can fall upwards. The Chinese news reports a stream where water flows up (See article below. 3-19-

2015).

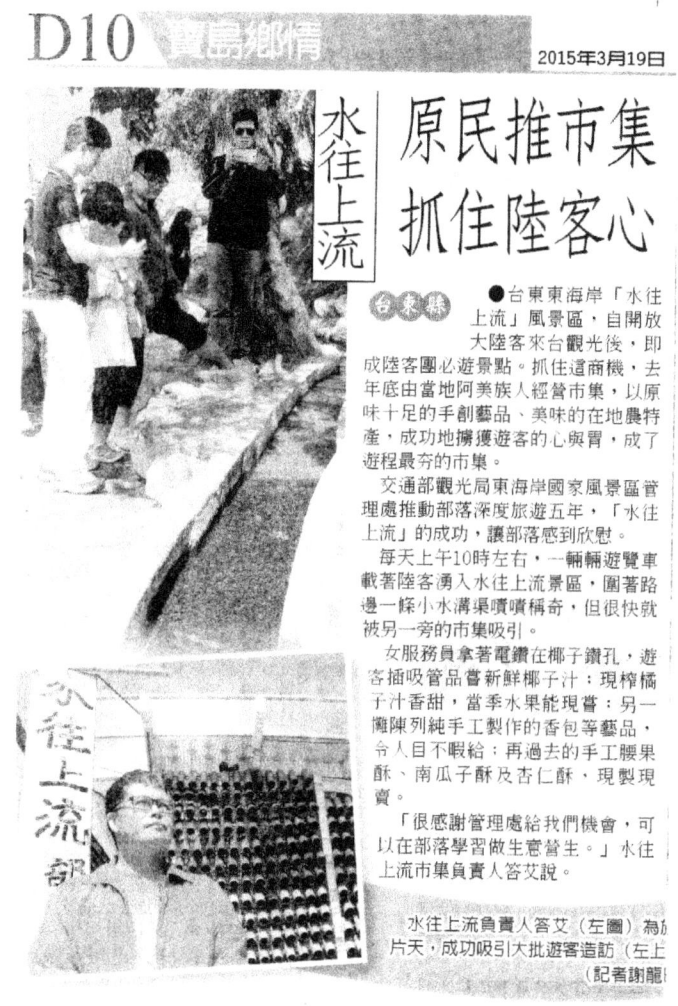

Figure 14

The newspaper article about water flowing up a stream in Taiwan.

But no Ph.D. is willing to spend the time to study the phenomena (maybe there are no funds for support). In a Chinese newspaper in 2013, the people even asked Dr. Young Zhen-Ning (Nobel prize in physics) about the phenomena, but he said he could not explain it.

But to the author, he is still studying it and some results point to "No Universal Gravity." If there was Universe Gravity, then Jesus being lifted to Heaven would be a liar. So as Enoch (Genesis 5:24) and Elijah (2 Kings 2:11). I also found the so-called "gravity" is actually another kind of force. And it is worth mentioning: that Malaysian Airlines Flight 370 (2014) had the accident because the airplane flew through the critical phase of the opposite "gravity." One side pulls down and the other side pulls up. This sheer force tore the airplane into two sections: one would fly high then drop and the other would fly down and far away from the front parts. This accident happened in Taiwan too. But nobody knew why the parts of the airplane were found in two groups. However, they were separated by a hundred miles. This phenomena also can be found at the Bermuda Triangle and the reason there are deserts with oasis in them.

Question #22 Can you prove that magnetic lines exist?
Answer: Again, here the author mentions the magnetic lines are actually Qi's line and nothing to do with magnetic lines. It only use that as a kind of model to explain in order to understand the Qi's line when in meridians that can only be through acupuncture points chart to see it, but they are still invisible. And those acupuncture points can not be seen either. Only until the author had one LUPUS patient. She is the most valuable living specimen with sixteen meridian, all sick— and that caused her whole body to have sores. The author found those sores are all located on the acupuncture points and those points can be connected as a meridian line as the acupuncture charts show.

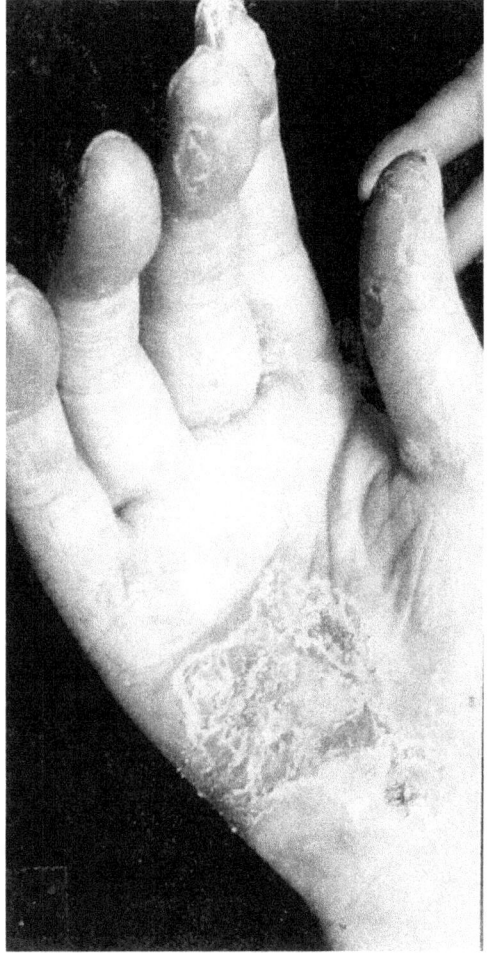

Figure 15

Right hand before treatment

The thumb means the lung and its meridian have problems. The second finger means the large intestine and its meridian have problems. The third finger means the pericardium and its meridians have problems. The fourth finger means triple warmers (three sections of the body except organs). The small finger means the heart and its meridians have problems.

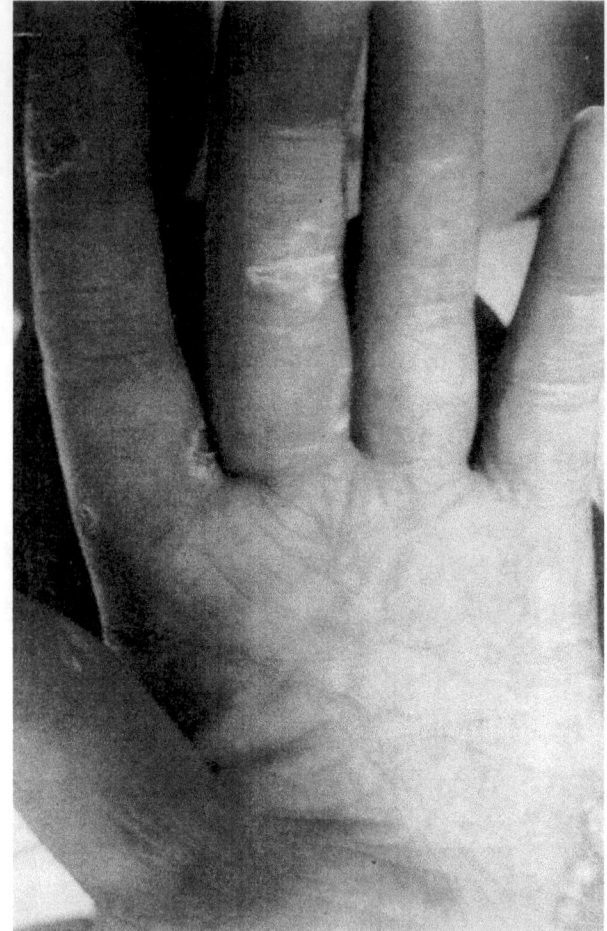

Figure 16

Left hand before treatment

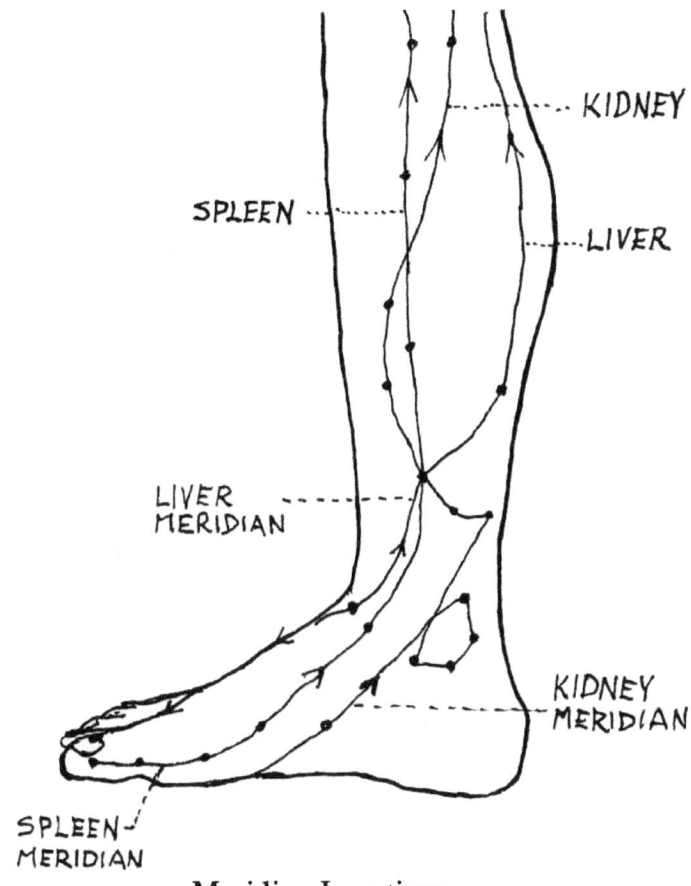

Meridian Locations

Figure 17

1…Since November 2009, I found the patient's right leg had a big sore. The hospital did nothing and said this could not be cured. So, the author took the patient to a private doctor for surgery and to take my herbal medicine as well. Then the recovery is shown in the other pictures. Also, you can see her toenails, half no good (was sick). Half became normal (after recovery) to prove that her liver and spleen meridians were getting to normal. (This takes a long time.)

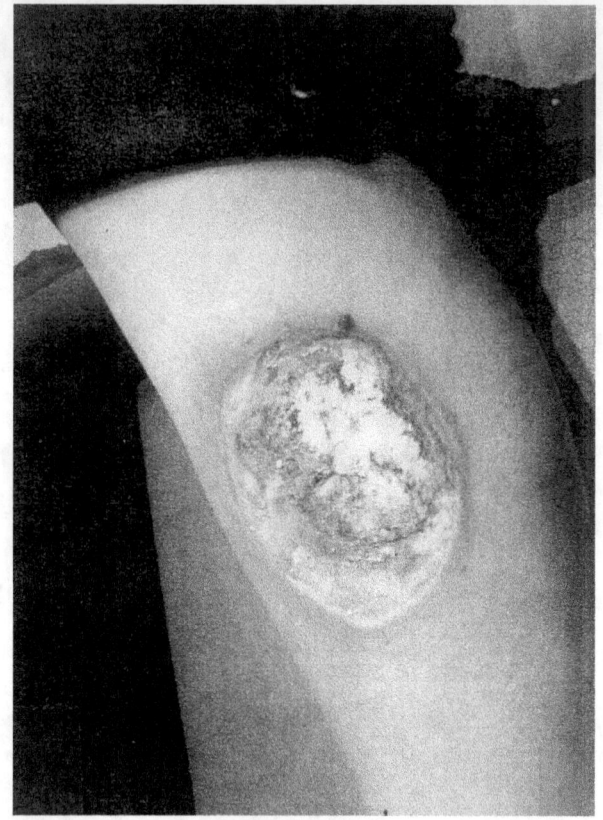

Figure 18

Before treatment

This big ulcer is located on the intersections of the spleen and kidney meridians.

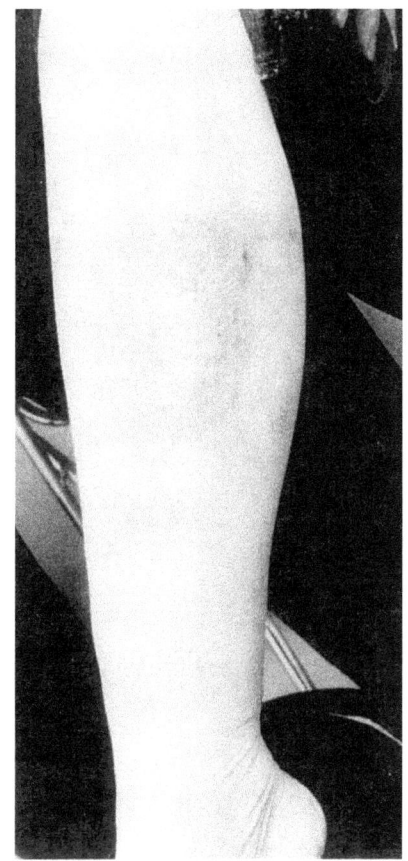

Figure 19

After treatment

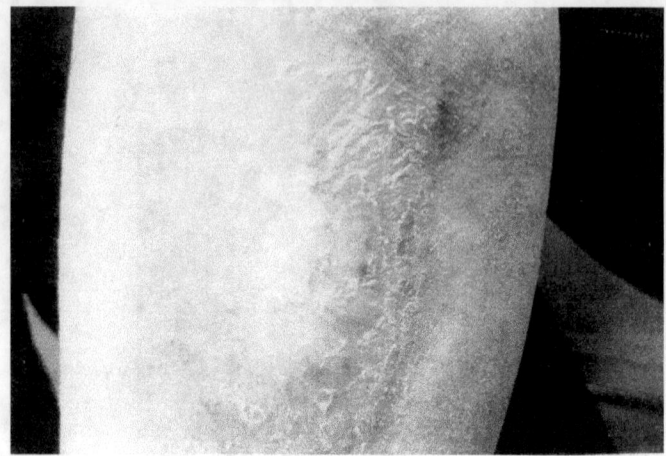

Figure 20

After treatment

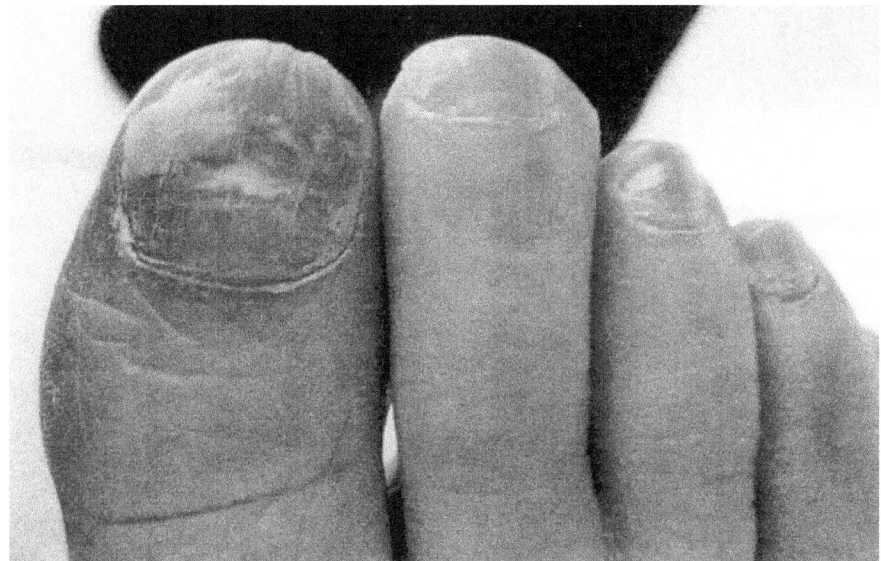

Figure 21

Left side of the toenail is cracked which means her spleen meridian
has dry blood inside. That will cause the nail of the sick toe to crack.
After treatment, the half section of new growth restored to its
original health.

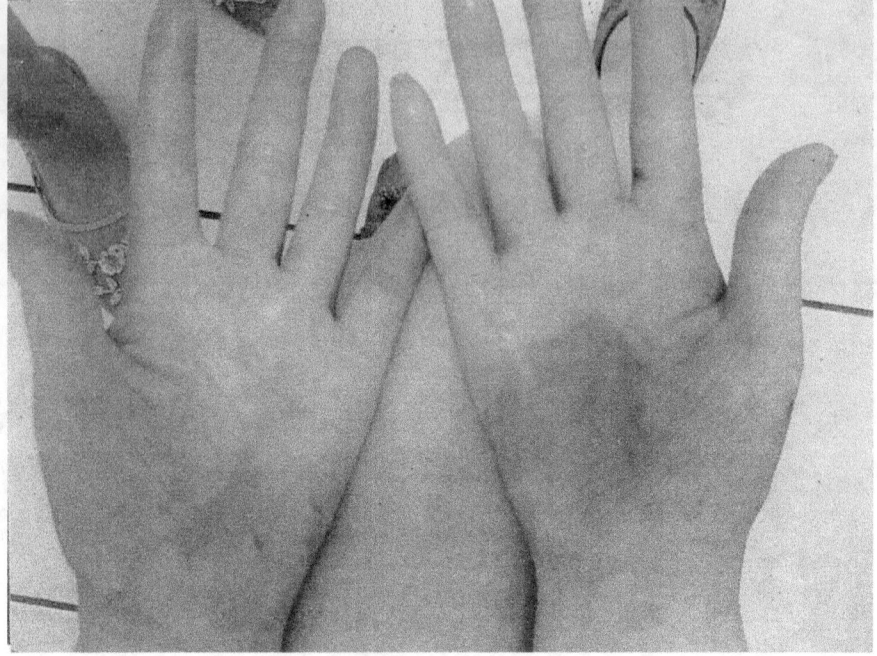

Figure 22

Two hands recovered after treatment

2…So as the hands

I have her picture of the whole body to match with the charts. Seeing the pictures will help people to believe. Also, one other example: if you go to check the picture of breast cancer, those cancer tumors are also located on the lower side and outer edge of the breast, and those tumors match the chart. They are located on the spleen meridian (line). That means the breast's cancer originally comes from the spleen. And those problems (such as upset, angry, and anxious) cause the illness and could not be relieved for years. That emotion will hurt the spleen (stated in the Chinese medical book). And from this picture of breast cancer, we can see what the book says is true. That is why Chinese common words say "get angry" is "produce spleen Qi."

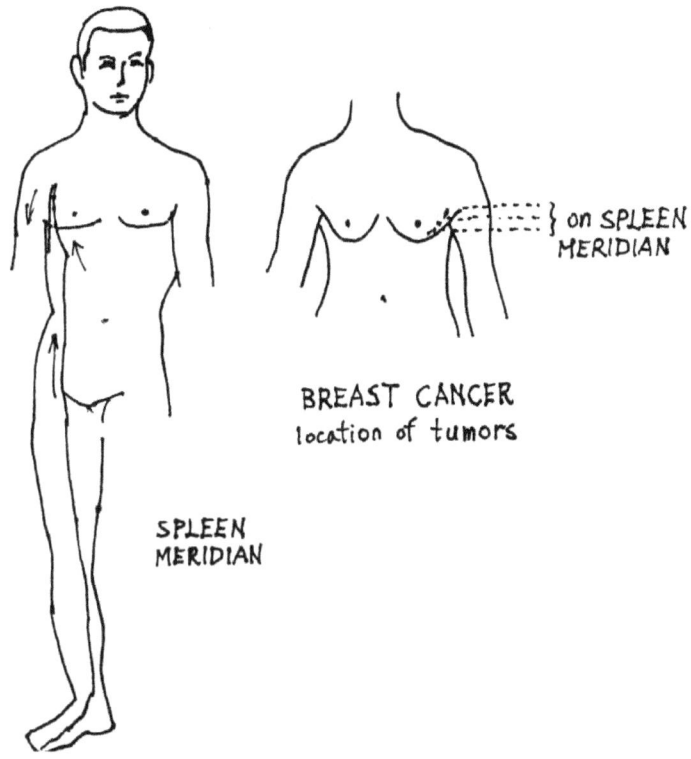

BREAST CANCER
location of tumors

} on SPLEEN
MERIDIAN

SPLEEN
MERIDIAN

Figure 23

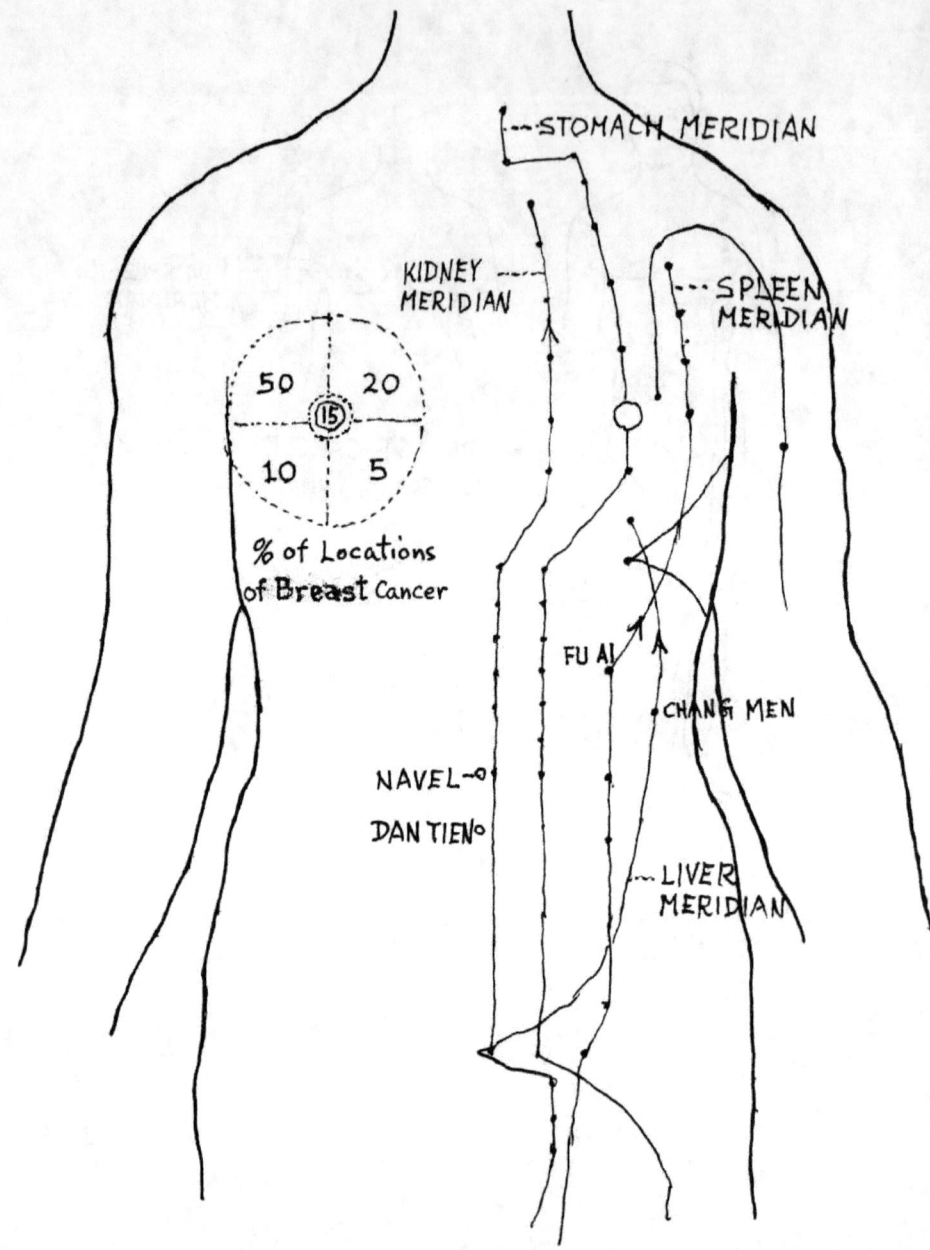

Figure 24
Detail Body Meridians
To produce Breast Cancer

Question #23 This is a belief that cannot be measured.

Answer: Fatigue cannot be measured. The analogy is a car: When the battery is weak, the driver would not know until the engine's starter cannot crank. People have to pay more attention: he will find that he feels tired easily after 8 hours of work and then feels the need to rest. But some people may feel tired six or even four hours. On the other hand, some people still feel tired after eight hours of rest.

Question #24 Parkinson's Disease is a neurological disease in the brain that causes loss of control of the bodily movements. Nerve diseases are not considered?

Answer: This is what the western doctor said. It is not true. As a matter of fact, Parkinson's is also caused from catch "wind," (usually we said catch a cold, but the cold comes in with the wind or air bubbles) into the meridian when the person is short of energy (overworked or oversexed), the author has had two cases (listed below).

a…One friend, who was the owner of a restaurant (located at 10 W 38th Street in New York City between 1990-2000), got Parkinson's due to overwork. Then he slept more (at least eight hours) and exercised a half hour more, and recovered within six months.
b…Another friend had a beautiful young wife (15 years younger). Later on, he developed Parkinson's (1995). I told him how to recover. Also, I wanted him to reduce his sexual activity. He said he would give up Viagra. After a few years, he had become hunchbacked, but his Parkinson's seemed improved. The Chinese medical textbook said: when wind (air bubbles) goes into the kidney, people become hunchbacked. In other words, the air bubbles flow from the meridian goes into the kidney so the Parkinson's gets better, but turned to hunchback. The western doctor said the hunchback was caused by his osseous tissue becoming fragile. And the real truth is air bubbles blocked the Qi to deliver calcium and nutrition to the

bone tissue.

Question #25 Blocked circulation will affect the hands and feet. Circulatory diseases are not considered, only magnetic explanation?
Answer: Just like the previous cases of Parkinson's and hunchbacked. Western doctors have a different explanation. But Chinese only said "wind" (air bubbles). Who is right? Actually, both are right. Just the western doctors measure the bone tissue test so it sounds more reliable for the results. On the other hand, the ancient Chinese doctors get the "Qi's" feeling of circulation that enables them to find the original causes even without any measurement tools or lab tests that western doctors use. That is why hundreds of diseases for western doctors don't know their causes. It turned out most diseases through the centuries still can only be under control, not cured.

Question #26 If homosexual couples are successful over many decades, does that mean their magnetic fields have not been damaged?
Answer: Like smoking, everybody knew that would cause lung cancer. But, a few people smoke a lot and live until age 90 or more. Their longevity depends on their health, living styles, sexual activity frequency and timing. Also, even though one of them is sick and dead. If they are a good partner (loyal to each other) and never overdo it, he might have died from pneumonia, yet the original reason of low energy level would not be of concern. This is the most difficult to define—the group with AIDS symptoms but no HIV virus and no cause alert for the medical professional. Especially, the survivor even could claim that he is gay (play the male role), but he is never sick from AIDS, so AIDS has nothing to do with homosexuality. That fact has confused the medical industry.

Question #27 What about any heterosexual couples who practice rectum intercourse who are not homosexuals? Are you saying that heterosexuals cannot live long lives? Why is there a problem with the magnetism because the rectum is on the other side of the vagina area?

Answer: This is a very interesting question. As the author's understanding, the heterosexual couples who practice rectum intercourse, there should be no such problem. His reason is that men's magnetic field (here should be emphasized Qi field, because the man's is called yang (positive) and different from women's Qi Field which is called ying (negative). So, even a man and woman who practice rectal intercourse, they would not have the expulsion happen. That is why the Bible only emphasized men and sounds like discrimination against women. This answer is totally the author's reasonable guess and indeed needs further proof.

Question # 28 Not sure if the delivery of a baby relates to vaginal intercourse?

Answer: This the author cannot answer, but only offer a reasonable guess. Later on, a friend of mine, Mr. Monroe, told me a story about his own experience. The author thinks this story may offer an answer:

My experience with gratification of sexual intercourse encounter that began with intimate foreplay involved all sensual faculties. Exploring all areas of my mate's body through touch and feel privileges, she reciprocated the same.

The interacting contact exchange between us escalated our desire in the act. Progressive stimulation triggered anticipation causing her vagina to contract and my penis as well. As I refrained from haste, I slowly inserted my instrument into her cleft of ecstasy while her vaginal contractions welcomed me.

I began winding in a moderate circular motion as I felt her vagina contractually "biting" my penis. My movement was complicated by the rhythm of her throwing her waist at me. Her legs embraced my waist in order to keep me close as she communicated through body language mixed with moans and groans that kept me penetrating her intermittently seeking the accelerated rhythm of her contractions mixed with mine until we both accomplished climax.

Also, the other friend, Mr. Thomas, taught me that:

1...Dr. Kegel's Exercise (for women's sexual training)
2...Brazil: Zumba dancing
3...Kama Sutra (India book, 2,500 years ago - *Secrets of Making Love*)
The engraved figures and pictures of making love shown in temples were based on this book.
There are more references the readers can find.

Question #29 Sperm is possible the body's battery electrical fluid?
Answer: In science, when we try to describe something new that never be defined before, usually we find an existing similar model to describe. For example: we describe sound, light, electric, electronic—all use water wave to describe these in order to be understandable. But maybe a little different. However, that won't influence the character we need to use

Question #30 The timing may not be a supported idea.
Answer: What the author means: because the semen is only a little volume and is concentrated in one area, not like blood which is throughout the body.

Question #31 What is the close relationship between saliva and sperm?
Answer: That means one's volume influences each other's volume. If you have lots of saliva, that can be seen when your sperm volume is full. The typical case is with babies: their saliva always overflow. That is why they need bibs all the time.

Question #32 Thirsty from heavy breathing that dried up the saliva?
Answer: The reason of thirst seems due to sexual exercise, but actually is different: regular thirst from exercise will be easily stopped by drinking a large glass of water. But, if from sexual activity, it seems it will be hard to stop the thirst.

Question #33 Spitting saliva makes people tired?
Answer: Yes, the person feels no strength. Then, when feeling tired,

a person will likely have coffee or a cigarette in order to feel energized again. Beware because coffee, cigarettes, and drugs give only a temporary energy boost. Those things just melt your bone density and become "Qi." This is the reverse function of "Qi Gong." Also, shell fish, especially the oyster, will melt your bone density and become "sperm." This is a little different. That is why some men like to have sex many times at night. Besides the Viagra, they will eat a dozen raw oysters.

Question #34 The Qi channel is magnetic and cannot be seen?
Answer: The Qi's channels are called meridians. (They are in the body along and connected to the acupuncture points.) The meridians are full of Qi and blood in different percentages.

Question # 35 Why the last sentence, if the person is dead?
Answer: Because this is the most serious damage of AIDS, but just without symptoms. (No HIV virus, no apparent difference from normal people). So, they would be excluded from AIDS patients by doctors. And then the analysis of AIDS will be short the most significant part. As the author would expect, a few then would die from AIDS. It turned out they were dead, but the announcement just said: pneumonia or heart failure.

Question #36 Women catch AIDS in various ways
Answer: This part we already discussed very clearly in a previous question. But, if by electrical toys or infected by fluid contamination would be another story.

Question #37 People who don't believe in body magnetism will want statistical evidence of this.
Answer: The people who don't believe in body magnetism do not mean "magnetism not existence." They can only say they just do not have time to get proof or say they just emotionally reject the "Qi" concept and see that concept as a kind of witchcraft. But in this book, the author has already brought some evidence—including his

161

teacher, Dr. Lee's experimental report. The author's other teacher, Master Wang, Zue-Ting, has a video that shows how a paralytic patient (same as Dr. Stephen Hawking, English physicist) can be lead (not healed yet, but it will take months to be treated) by the Master's Qi and exercise as normal right away. Also, the news said so.

Question #38 The heart would be cold before 24 hours. Do the Chinese practice this today? Why don't the Chinese doctors tell the world? It seems like a big secret.

Answer: Those kinds of deaths usually are only caused from lack of oxygen, then the heart stops. Just like a mobile car, you turn off the engine does not mean the battery is dead. This is similar to those animals who can hibernate. Therefore, the heart may be cold before 24 hours, but may not be that hard, because the energy Qi will still give the organs heat, even without blood circulation. The author does not think the Chinese practice that today: because the people who know the recent Chinese history over the past century, then that person will understand through at least ten big wars (including WWI and WWII), especially under the Japanese invasion, ruffian, the Chinese civil war, and cultural revolution. Everything seems lost, only you can get from a few old books which are not popular with the medical industry or even said as no statistical proof. So, because of no weight in school and society, it seems like witchcraft, rather than a big secret, especially involved with "Qi Gong"—because invisible, could not be proved, even the most practical techniques, such as acupuncture, are not accepted by the medical industry until President Nixon went to China in 1960. Like the author, he has been trying to introduce all this special knowledge to Americans. It has taken thirty years to get enough proof to publish this book, even without any financial support, plus all kinds of legal barriers and medical industry barriers. That is why so much troubles are in western society. One important reason: all the medical system is following the western system during the past century. So, the Chinese doctors who are handling the administration of the medical industry are all educated by western medical schools. They become the same as the western doctors, but short of oriental medical knowledge. Also, there had not been an oriental medical school in China until 1970. In the civil market, only the traditional Master-disciples system still exists.

Question #39 Avoiding masturbation needs further explanation as a reminder.
Answer: The explanation has already been given. The author could not provide some further proof due to the privacy of the case.

Question #40 We know some cancer causes. Example, skin cancer from too much sun exposure.
Answer: That is right to say such as skin cancer from too much sun exposure, or lung cancer from too much smoke. But still, not everyone under the same conditions would get cancer. But why? Or some patients not even get sunburned or smoke, they still get sick. So, the real causes still need to be studied. But overall, the stronger ones still can prevent suffering (not muscle strong, but Qi or energy strong).

Question #41 Radiation and chemo can work on some cancers
Answer: Radiation can burn and kill the cancer cells. But these are not really the way to treat the cancers. That is why, after these procedures, they still have to wait five years to see if the cancers come back. And most of the time, they come back. That's what makes the cancers so scary to everybody. And according to the author's discovery and treatment, the real causes are: <u>fever from air bubbles caused or being upset or angry in the tissues or organs, for a little period will mix the moisture and then produce the toxin. So, the cancer cells are beginning to produce.</u> (Blood cancer or leukemia is different and an exception: that is a "cold" in the "kidneys," so the focus should be on the kidney instead of the bone marrow, but doctors don't know that.)

And the treatment of that:

Fever: western doctors can only use drugs such as Prednisone. However, these steroids can only separate antigen and antibody, but cannot stop the production of antigens. Because the fever is produced all the time. And the fever was originally produced due to the air bubble staying in the meridian that causes fever when Qi passes through it. "Rub, friction produce heat in physics." That is why, until a certain period, the fever will be out of control. Even high doses of Prednison could not bring down the fever.

Moisture: western doctors totally neglect this because in the lab experiments, moisture is never a concern.

Toxin: So far, western medicine cannot solve this problem that causes severe pain for which painkillers do not even work. Even the "radiation" could not burn the toxin. If you study the Chinese Herbal Medical book, there are ways to treat disease by burning the herbs and their ash can still be used, because their character does not disappear.

These are the author's personal results and he will write about in more detail in his next book—LUPUS *and My Million Dollar Patient.*

As for the author's LUPUS patient, her western doctors kept asking her about some symptoms that doctors assumed cancer was going to happen in her body. But it never happened. Actually, it happened, but the author treated it with herbs right away and it worked.

One exception is leukemia (blood cancer). That is "cold" in the kidney that makes the white blood cells keep on being produced. That is opposite to LUPUS, which makes the white blood cells reduce. The western doctors treat blood cancer by exchanging bone marrow and chemotherapy which is too complicated and too costly. As long as they remove the "cold," the white blood cells will be reduced automatically. That is another example: doctors thought of blood made from bone marrow, but they did not know bone marrow is handled by the kidneys. That is why after changed bone marrow, patients still mostly died.

Question #42 Drugs exist that extend the lives of AIDS patients. **Answer:** Yes, after 30 years of effort, the cocktail treatment for AIDS seems to have worked. But that is only under control for some types of AIDS patients. The patients have to take medicine all their lives. Because the original cause was not found yet. That means the drugs have not really worked. Also, many AIDS patients died because their sickness was out of control. Just like LUPUS patients, they were given "Prednisone," but some patients still died from "high fever" that could not be brought down by Prednisone. This is something the doctors cannot deny.

Question #43 How can you prove what you say?
Answer: This cannot be proved because "data" cannot be established. Just like acupuncture, to get permission in the American medical industry, there is no cooperation. Thus, there is no data to show the public, administrators, and senators to get their affirmation. But all the acupuncture doctors, when using the needle, they have a feeling about:

1...got Qi when they have the right point and the right depth. (some of the point needle need to be half inch, some one inch, some two inches...the feeling is a little like electric shock when the needle pierces into the skin at the right point and the right depth.

2...when turned right, we give energy to the patient at that point.

3...when turned left, we replenish the energy out from that point.

So as the patients:

1...they will feel the minor electric shock first.

2...the shock feeling will extend along the Meridian from point to point, and that point will have a pumping-like pulse.

3...Sometimes, even be influential at the ends of the Meridian or its company of that Meridian. (In the body, there are 6 pairs of Meridian, such as (1) heart and small intestines, (2) lung and large intestines, (3) kidney and urine bladder, (4) spleen and stomach, and (5) liver and gallbladder, and (6) triple warmer and pericardium. Note: Triple warmer is a term that contains the Upper part (chest), Middle part (about the stomach location), and Lower part (below the belly button). It is not an organ. But it seems to contain the whole body, except the organs. It is also strange and makes the author wonder that the system has triple warmer as an organ, but neglects the existence of the pancreas.

4…when the needle is turned left, the patient will feel relief of swelling and pain

5…when the needle is turned to the right, the patient will feel the energy come in from the needle.

Question #44 The time length may be incorrect.
Answer: That is right, because no tools can measure how much energy still is in the tissue or sphere field. Another example: When people are being beheaded, the head was separated from the body, but the eyes are still winking and the hands or legs will still seized.

Question #45 The term does not mean anything to someone not trained.
Answer: If people want to learn, they must know this term and it is one important function of Qi Gong. It is typical for helping men's swollen prostate. Also, there is an important concept here: unobstructed (passing through) then is no pain, but obstructed then is pain. And obstructions are caused by Qi, air bubbles, moisture, toxins, and cracks or splits, heat, freeze, etc.

Question #46 Genetic and bad genes are reasons for deformities.
Answers: Generally speaking, that is right. But marriages of close relative seem to have more chances than non-relatives marrying (different last names), according to statistics. A long time ago, the author had a friend who did his graduate essay to research the Jewish genetics probably for that reason of intermarriages.

Question #47 Further, to be a geomancer, astrologer or prophet.
Answer: Geomancer: In China, the geomancer when he goes any place, he can feel the "Qi" of the environment, such as when the Qi is too sharp (like a knife), too suffocating, too cold, too open, too gloomy, and so on. So not only that, he will suggest how to arrange

the furniture, mirror, trees, water pond, entrance, and so on. But also he will use a compass to measure in case his feelings are not correct. And one very interesting thing: the compass does not always point north in some places. That means the earth's magnetic field is abnormal or unclean. In this point, the Amish people who do not use electric devices may have their good reasons.

Astrologer: the one who watches the stars and who can tell the fortune of governments or other important subjects. The author does not know about astrology, except through fiction books. But in the Bible: three wise men went to look for Jesus through the leading of a star. Sounds similar. Besides that, the author has a few friends who can see ghosts in the lamplight. Also, some of them can calculate something to tell your fortune and in the future, and reveal your past dates. The author met them in Dr. Qing-Tse Lee's class.

Prophet: (1) Some of these people were born to be prophets; (2) some of them were through the special method and get their power from ghosts (good or bad). The examples are: the Live Buda (he made that claim himself – Lu, Sen-Yen from Division of true Buddhism, the Master Lee, Hong-Zhi from FaLun Da Fa (these two are still alive), the Prophet Elisha from Elijah (I Kings 19:16) whose power was from God.; and (3) some of them have power through practice and obtaining the ability. As the author mentioned before, the levels of Regular Eyes (or Flesh Eyes), Heavenly Eye, Deva Eye, Propaganda Eye, and Buddha's Eye. Lots of books said that, but in Fa LunDaFa (from Internet), the methods and phenomena have been described very clearly.

Question #48 All knowledge?
Answer: Food (whether good or bad for health), herbs, medical diagnosis and treatments, religions, geomancy, fortunetelling, martial arts, and even common language are full of the terms of Qi Gong. People used it all the time, but did not know it.

Question #49 Heaven and Hell concepts, which developed in India and China, were based on ancient Egypt?

Answer: The author does not know much about Egypt. In China and India, many spiritual mediums could bring people to heaven or hell to look for their relatives. And, meanwhile, they could see what activities were taking place in Heaven or Hell. We all know that King Saul had asked a familiar spirit to get Prophet Samuel's spirit out from death (I Samuel 28:4-25). That means they already knew the concept of Heavan and Hell in ancient Egypt, but they were not clear how that related to Qi Gong.

Deuteronomy 18:9-14: "When you come into the land that the Lord your God is giving you, don't follow the disgusting practices of the nations that are there. Don't sacrifice your children in the fires on your altars; and don't let your people practice divination or look for omens or use spells or charms and don't let them consult the spirits of the dead. The Lord your God hates people who do these disgusting things, and that is why he is driving those nations out of the land as you advance. Be completely faithful to the Lord. Then Moses said, "In the land you are about to occupy, people follow the advice of those who practice divination and look for omens, but the Lord your God does not allow you to do this. Instead, he will send you a prophet like me from among your own people, and you are to obey him."

This is the fact that in western culture, except for God, everything seems evil.

In I Samuel 28:4-19, it is written:

"The Philistine troops assembled and camped near the town of Shunem. Saul gathered the Israelites and camped at Mount Gilboa. When Saul saw the Philistine army, he was terrified, and so he asked the Lord what to do. But the Lord did not answer him at all, either by dreams or by the use of Urim and Thummim or by prophets. Then Saul ordered his officials, 'Find me a woman who is a medium and I will go and consult with her.' 'There is one in Endor,' they answered. So Saul disguised himself, he put on different clothes, and after dark he went with two of his men to see the woman. 'Consult the spirits for me and tell me what is going to happen,' he said to her. 'Call up the spirit of the man I name.' The woman answered, "Surely you know what King Saul has done, how he forced the fortunetellers and mediums to leave Israel. Why, then, are you trying to trap me and get me killed?' Then Saul made a sacred vow. 'By the living Lord, I promise that you will not be punished for doing this,'' he told her. 'Whom shall I call up for you?' the woman asked. 'Samuel,' he answered. When the woman saw Samuel, she screamed and said to Saul, 'Why have you tricked me? You are King Saul.' 'Don't be afraid.' the king said to her. 'What do you see?' 'I see a spirit coming up from the earth,' she answered. 'He is wearing a cloak.' Then Saul knew that it was Samuel and he bowed to the ground in respect. Samuel said to Saul, 'Why have you disturbed me? Why did you make me come back?' Saul answered, 'I am in great trouble. The Philistines are at war with me. And God has abandoned me. He doesn't answer me anymore, either by prophets or by dreams. And so I have called you, for you to tell me what I must do.' Samuel said, 'Why do you call me when the Lord has abandoned you and become your enemy? The Lord has done to you what he told you through me: he has taken the kingdom away from you and given it to David instead. You disobeyed the Lord's command and did not completely destroy the Amalekites and all they had. That is why the Lord is doing this to you now. He will give you and Israel over to the Philistines. Tomorrow you and your sons will join me, and the Lord will also give the army of Israel over to the Philistines."

From this story, we can see and summarize:

(1)…Under Christianity, to learn or to practice those techniques involved with the spirit are prohibited and not even to be studied as to how they work—so it became lost and thought of as fiction.

(2)…This technique really works to call the spirit back: (a) even though Samuel was a great prophet who belonged to God, it seems he could not ignore her calling; (b) people can communicate with the spirits of the dead; and the spirit of the dead person knows a lot of things that are going to happen in the future.

If you believe in the Bible, you should not deny this. Then many similar cases in oriental religious division, their existing miracles should be given credit too. So as "How it works"—which is based on

"Qi," should be given credit too.

For example: In Taiwan, Taoism, very popular for a specialty to communicate the death and the lives for people, but one time the author's grandfather experienced that when he was there, the witchcraft (Gi-Tong) could not function; then the Gi-Tong asked, "who is believer of western religion? Please leave here! Otherwise, my sorcery cannot work." This case made grandpa very proud of being a Christian.

The other example: One pastor, Mr. Tong, who was the son of a sorcerer of Taiwanese native Indian. Since he changed his religion, he asked his father to follow him. Very struggled and confused, it ended up the father (sorcerer) had to perform sorcery to ask their god. Very surprisingly their God told the father that Jesus is greater than their god, and their family had no problem to change their religion. (Note: That means their god is a good God too and so we understand that in the Bible: God Jehovah put Jewish only (actually only Abraham and his family) under his own jurisdiction. Other races have their own guardian angels (Gods).

Question #50 Hard to understand how wanting a king relates to Qi Gong.
Answer: Wanting a king means rejecting the governance of God. Just like asking fortunetellers and mediums for advice, instead of praying to God.

Since Rome's empire legalized the Catholic Church as a national religion, fortunetellers and mediums became illegal and fiction for thousands of years. They end up "the why and how it worked." Nobody goes for further study and research anymore. That is how western society seems to have no idea about "Qi." Because most good religions when they communicate with their gods, the way the sorcerer performed is related to "Qi."

Also, people still confused the difference between a prophet and a medium, even a good prophet from a bad prophet.

Question #51: Wikipedia: magnetic field in humans does not exist as a topic.

Answer: Please look at the article from Agence France Presse (Dec 29, 2013) where a man can attract 53 pieces of soup spoons. That means humans do have magnetic fields, only most people cannot develop it (Question #4).

Question #52: An article in *Real Health* (Fall, 2013) reports better cures and remissions for HIV (AIDS) if the antiretroviral medications are given as soon as possible, including remission in infants who have been treated early.

1…What is your reaction to the early use of medications for curing HIV (AIDS)?

Answer: The author comments: Diseases from bacteria, viruses, and antigens—those can get better cures and remissions if the medications are given in time because our own immune system was not damaged yet. But differences between cure and remissions depend on acquiring from infection or producing from the patient's own body. If from the patient's own body, then only remission for a little while; the disease will come again. That obviously happened on the LUPUS patient's body too. So, it ends up out of control. So as all kinds of cancers can be out of control. <u>Because the real "causes" are not studied by the doctors.</u> <u>The doctors' medications are based on "dead tissue" in the laboratory.</u>

Question #53: What importance does Qi have, if any, in treating infants or children who are not able to use Qi techniques?

Answer: Please look at Chapter 12 (b) the faction of "Nei Jin Yi Zhi Chan." Their masters can use their Qi to treat patients. Check the internet, even "polio" that can be cured. If you check the Internet, their website will be clear. So do the author's teachers: Dr. Lee, Qing-tse and Master Sen, Hong-Shun (Tai Chi Wu Syn Gong). Also, it is necessary to take herbal ginseng tea as an option. However, it should be taken this way:

a…Don't cook in a metal pot because the "Qi" of ginseng may be attracted by the pot, which will reduce its efficiency.

 b…The dose of ginseng (dried root):

   1…Korean Ginseng or Chinese North-Eastern Ginseng: 5 grams each time.

   2…Others include: Dang Seng; American Ginseng; Sah Seng; Tai-Ze Seng: 15-20

  grams each time.

   3…Take 2-3 times a day.

 c…Don't eat peanuts while you are taking ginseng.

 d…Don't eat radish or turnip at the same time.

Question #54: Even though you have already had a few cases to show that you could really cure what the Western doctors cannot, according to regulations, without massive numbers of cases to prove, all that you have shown are not countable.

Answer: The author is an engineer. We all know that the creation of machines, once the idea is correct, then from the research to the solid creation not too many experiments are needed. Contrarily, if the concept is not appropriate, although there were thousands of cases to prove, it turns out there will be failure. That is, how many medicines were taken off the market because of the dangers of their side effects. Besides, the author has already pointed out: most medicine was studied in the laboratory on dead tissue and neglected the patients' bodies. (The living environment includes antigens, viruses, cancer cells, bacteria, and so on.) Both doctors and patients did not know that even without that specific medicine the side effects would be happening anyway.

Question #55: You keep on saying that Western doctors did not study the herbal treatments and governments did not make any efforts to help. Don't you know that we have the official the National Center of Complementary and Integrative Health (NCCIH) that offers plenty of funding for research?

Answer: Obviously, NO herbal treatment in any hospital or by any doctor is covered by an insurance policy. NCCIH requires the applicants to be treated by the western methods and those with western diplomas. However, because of these requirements, all of them will present the same mistakes: (a) study the dead tissue; (b) have no idea about Qi Gong—energy system which is totally absent from western anatomy; (c) have no idea about fever, chills, moisture, dryness, toxins, wind, and so on that are the real causes of illnesses and diseases; and Western doctors totally ignore the knowledge of the oriental medical system, which include herbal compound formulas and oriental pathologies that have been established already for thousands of years. So, even though NCCIH has been established for a long time, the really good results are still only limited.

Question #56: You complained that doctors and government did not do this or do that. It sounds like they are all bad guys in spite of whatever good results they have already acquired. If you had authority, what are you going to do and what can you develop further?

Answer: Within one year, I will have at least ten kinds of herbal medicines through three testing phases required by the FDA, and on the market and in hospitals to supplement the insufficient western medicines, such as (a) the fever that Prednisone could not control that I rescued the patient in Missouri as already shown in the book; (b) the pain of cancer that morphine cannot stop, a pain due to a toxin; (c) the medicine for Mesothelioma; (d) the medicine to cure leukemia (reduce WBC): If I could increase WBC for LUPUS patients, to reduce should be no problem, only reverse the way. And arthritis medicines (about 10 different kinds according to the locations of pain in the body). Furthermore, these formulas will be well open to the public without a patent enabling the pharmacists to use them along with western medicines and then refine as ACT (which just got the Nobel prize) because the techniques of western medicine are well developed after all.

All the doctors will need to learn Qi Gong for three months (total of 100 hours), so the discussion of the energy system will be practical.

Real energy medicine will be on the market, instead of cigarettes, coffee, or other stimulants such as the caffeine-based Red Bull drink. When people need to work longer or harder, they will not be hurting themselves. (This can be of special help for doctors who work long hours.)

If my advice continues to be ignored by the U.S. government, then I believe that Taiwan, Hong Kong, China, Japan, and Korea will go ahead and execute my ideas. I believe this because I believe there is a medical revolution coming:

Treatment costs: my treatment would be thousands of dollars, not hundreds of thousands

Treatment periods: my treatments would be months, not years

Medicines: new ones provided in an efficiently and in a short period (within one year) compared to the existing long-term testing period today (10 years).

Costs: my medicines would be much more affordable compared to today's prices.

Question #57: You seemed to try to say that you are the one who was predicted in the Bible where it says "the stone which the builders (peers) rejected (thought it useless), has become the head of the corner" (Psalm 118:22-23). Do you know that Jesus had cited these verses to himself already (Matthew 21:42; Mark12:10-11), so the disciples applied it to Jesus (Acts 4:11; Ephesians 2:20; 1st Philippians 2:7). How dare you try to grab His glory and say Jesus was ever wrong.

Answer:

First, Jesus had been wrong (Matthew 12:32) in a few places in the Bible: Jesus said that the end of the world will happen before the people then living had all died (Mark 13:30, Matthew 16:23), so it looks like He could be that one.

But in fact: (1) the end of the world did not happen even after 2000 years. (2) Jesus had never been seen as useless, but as a healer, miracle performer, the Evil One who offended God's laws (Matthew 10: 24-25; Matthew 9:3, 34; Matthew 12:22-30; Matthew 15:10-20; Matthew 27: 37, 40; Mark 3:30). (3) There are many cornerstones, however, the foundation Rock is Peter, while the great stone which hit the giant statutes and shattered them is Jesus (Daniel 2:34-35; Matthew 22:44). Second, the one seen as the useless stone, or like the Chinese said, "Decayed wood cannot be carved" is the author: when he was 57, he tried to be trained in a free-tuition nursing program and was rejected because his English score was lower than 40% of the competitors in spite of his math score at 99%.

Third, verse 23: this is the Lord's doing, it is marvelous in our eyes; verse 24: this is the day which the Lord has made, we will rejoice and be glad in it. In Jesus' time, nobody rejoiced and was glad in it, even His disciples were scared and ran away. Of course, nobody felt marvelous either.

Today only: A cleaner (author) not only rescued a LUPUS patient from a situation in the emergency room where the doctors said there was no hope, but also cured her within three months, all remotely. Furthermore, he pointed out all the mistakes of the medical profession with evidence and that is called "marvelous."

APPENDIX A

AIDS Update News

AIDS update news digest from: *Chinese World Journal* 12-21, 2014
Author: Dr. Gi-Der Chang, Digest and translated by Mingguo Cho.

1...CDC estimates: there are 1.2 million (HIV/AIDS) patients.
2...50,000 newly infected patients annually (Male:Female = 4:1).
3...80% of male patients are gay.
4...20% of gays are AIDS patients.
5...The number of patients dying from AIDS total more than 650,000 so far, and more than 50% of them are gays.
6...Essays about AIDS total more than 10,000 pieces.
7...Money spent on AIDS by the U.S. government and private funds total more than one hundred billion in the past 30 years.
8...Most AIDS patients, because they have a weakened immune system, also have TB, cancers, and meningitis that showed up first in their bodies. Until then, patients were found to have had AIDS. (Typical AIDS symptoms happened first, then an illness of another disease, and finally HIV.) Exactly as the author predicted 25 years ago.
9...During 2012, the CDC estimated:
a...$23,000 annually was the medical cost for treating an AIDS patient.
b...$380,000 was the total cost per AIDS patient before they died.
c...Consider that there are 1.2 million AIDS patients out there now. Can we afford to treat these patients without finding better treatments with Qi Gong?

APPENDIX B

FALUN GONG BROCHURE

An Ancient Practice for A Modern Age

What Practicing Falun Gong Means to Me

Falun Gong gives me the knowledge and wisdom to be a better son, husband and friend. It allows me to make the right choices even in difficult circumstances.
Nick, Phoenix

Falun Gong lifted my depression dramatically.
Tysan, New York

I used to suffer from chronic angina and gastroenteritis, but they completely disappeared once I started practicing Falun Gong.
Connie, London

Pretty much everyone in Beijing knew somebody who had tried it and benefitted, physically or psychologically.
Zhao Ming, former Beijing resident

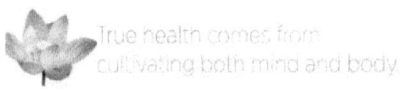 True health comes from cultivating both mind and body.

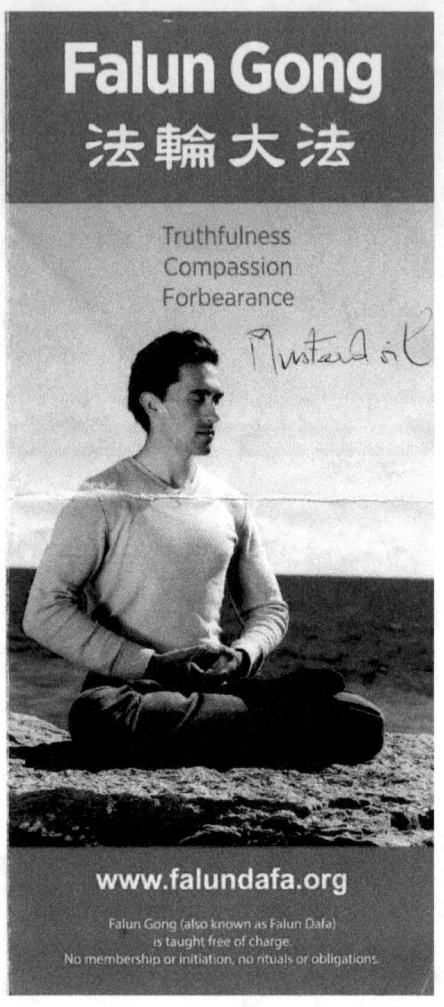

Falun Gong
法輪大法

Truthfulness
Compassion
Forbearance

www.falundafa.org

Falun Gong (also known as Falun Dafa) is taught free of charge. No membership or initiation, no rituals or obligations.

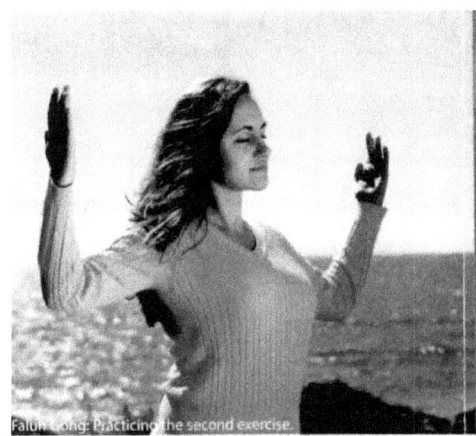

Falun Gong: Practicing the second exercise.

> Falun Gong is, in my judgement, the greatest single spiritual movement in Asia today. There is nothing that begins to compare with it in courage and importance.

Mark Palmer, former U.S. Ambassador to Hungary and Vice Chairman of Freedom House

Three Simple Ways to Start Learning:

1. Stop by a local practice site to learn the Falun Gong exercises. All Falun Gong exercise instructions are free of charge.

2. Read the teachings online: www.FalunDafa.org.

3. Learn the exercises from the Falun Dafa exercise instruction video and watch the 9-session lecture given by Mr. Li Hongzhi, the founder of Falun Dafa.

Millions Wrongly Persecuted in China Even Today

- 100 million people were practicing Falun Gong when the persecution began in 1999.

- Millions of Chinese people have since been abducted, imprisoned, tortured, fired from jobs, expelled from school, or forced into homelessness because they practice Falun Gong.

- Over 80,000 cases of torture have been recorded on www.minghui.org.

- Thousands have been killed.

Two Simple Things You Can Do to Help:

- Give this flyer to someone you know.

- Sign a petition at fofg.org.

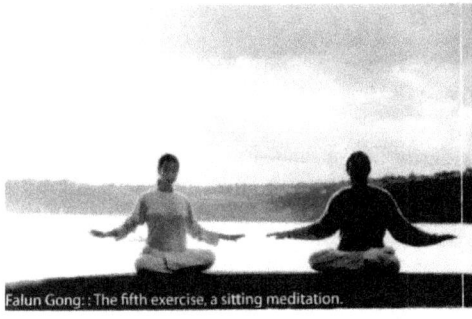

Falun Gong: : The fifth exercise, a sitting meditation.

The Five Exercises of Falun Dafa:

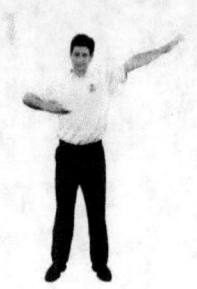 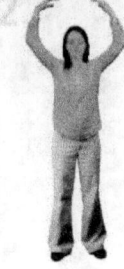 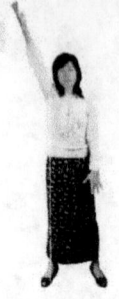 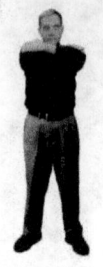 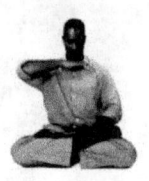

Buddha Displaying a Thousand Hands
Using gentle stretching movements, the first exercise opens all of the body's energy channels, creating a powerful energy field.

Falun Standing Stance
Comprised of four still positions that can be held for several minutes each, the second exercise boosts energy levels and awakens wisdom.

Penetrating the Two Extremes
With its gentle hand-gliding movements, the third exercise purifies the body using energy from the cosmos.

Falun Cosmic Circuit
By gently tracing the hands over the body, front and back, the fourth exercise rectifies abnormal conditions in the body and circulates energy.

Strengthening Higher Abilities
A meditation that incorporates special mudra and hand positions to refine body and mind, the fifth exercise strengthens higher abilities and energy.

The Teachings of Falun Dafa:

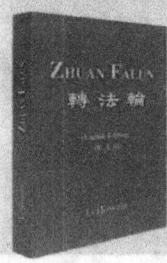

The book *Zhuan Falun (Revolving the Law Wheel)* by Mr. Li Hongzhi is the most comprehensive and essential set of teachings in the practice.

Falun Gong is an introductory text recommended for beginners. These and other works have been translated into thirty-eight languages.

All of Mr. Li's writings, as well as video instructions of Falun Dafa's exercises, can be downloaded for free at:
www.Falundafa.org

Books can also be purchased online by visiting www.Tiantibooks.org
Tel: +1 201 897 8788

ABOUT THE AUTHOR

MINGGUO CHO was born in Taiwan in 1948. He graduated with Architecture Engineering B.A. degree. After two years military service as a nurse, he came to the United States and became a naturalized citizen in 1982. For thirty years, he has studied and self-taught himself, besides work experience. Some studies include: Qi gong, Martial Arts, Acupuncture, Acupressure, Chinese Herbal Medicine, West Medical System (medicine, treatment methods, lab reports), diseases (AIDS, lupus, tumors) and Car Repairing.

This book explains his understanding and discoveries about the differences between Chinese ancient medical system and contemporary western medical system. The major difference is the Energy (Qi) system is totally absent from the anatomy, because they are invisible. Only through the practice of Qi gong can people feel it. However, that is how AIDS, Alzheimer's, and Multiple Sclerosis were developed. As a layman, he actually proved with medical report evidence and doctors as witnesses that he is completely correct. Most horrible disease become curable because the causes are clearly found.

ADDITIONAL BACKGROUND PROVIDED BY THE AUTHOR

1…Architecture Engineer background

2…Nurse in Taiwanese Army

3…Self-studied

Subjects: Herbs, Qi Gong, Martial Arts, Acupuncture and Acupressure, car repairing DIV, and western medical system's medicine, treatment methods, and medical lab reports.

He combined this information to a brand new stage, including the whole picture of the Ancient Oriental medical system in order to point out what was wrong with the western medical system.

Not only that, based on these concepts, he actually cured a LUPUS patient in a critical situation. (She was abandoned by the doctors and 1,000 miles away from the author.)

Also, he trained an AIDS patient with Qi Gong from barely walking to becoming strong enough to going back to ESL school, and strong enough to have a girlfriend after three months.

4…The author accomplished many revolutionary concepts and discoveries as a layman, not only medical and physical, but also religious in scientific ways in order to prove what he found. He gives all the credit to his accomplishments to God's will.

5…For thirty years, the author has dedicated himself while using his own money and time to discover why certain diseases could not be cured. In the end, he accomplished his goal and found the cures.

6…The author believes that he can help save more lives than those who died in World War II. In addition, he proved the cures will help save the patients and the government billions of dollars.

7…The author's goal is to be awarded three Nobel prizes: Peace, Medical, and Physics.

8…By reading his book, the author believes readers will find what he has written the truth instead of imagination.

9…The author also has a professional website: **mingguoalternativehealing.com**. It shows his concern is not only focused on human health, but also on animals and plagues.

Isaiah 29:14: Therefore behold, I will again do marvelous things with this people, wonderful and marvelous; and the wisdom of their wise men shall perish, and the discernment of their discerning men shall be hid.

(So many diseases, the doctors could not even understand their causes, but they claimed they knew how the human being evolved; so many Ph.D.s don't know that "there is no universal gravity. The so-called gravity really comes from the magnet wave's density." And these Ph.D.s tried to tell us how the universe was formed.)

Psalm 118:22-23: The stone which the builders (peers) rejected, has become the head of the corner: (corner stones which connect right wall—east and left wall—west; also connect the bottom stones—anciency (ancient Chinese wisdom) and upper stone—contemporary and future.

This is the Lord's doing; it is marvelous in our eyes.

This is the day which the Lord has made, let us rejoice and be glad in it.

REPENT. WE ALL NEED TO.

02/05/2005: The author was rejected to be considered for the Board of Adult Practical Nursing Program to become a nurse when he was 57 years old.

Oct to Dec/2008: The author cured the LUPUS patient Jennifer L.

who was rejected for treatment and sent home from the Emergency Room at the University Hospital, Columbia, Missouri.

Before this day, Ms. Jennifer had been treated for five years (since February, 2004). Within three months, the author not only saved her from her emergency condition, but also cured her. There is a medical report as proof. Amazingly, the author and Ms. Jennifer never saw each other. The author was living in New York City and had never been to Missouri.

The witnesses: Dr. Darcy D. Folzenlogen, M.D.
          Dr. Michael Cooper Stock, M.D.

The Court Case: Attorney General of Missouri, Jefferson City, MO
Attorney General: Chris Koster/Complaint # CF-2009-05653
Date: July, 2009

THE END